ENT Head and Neck Surgery

Extended Matching Items

Dr Ricardo Persaud

FRCS ORL-HNS (Eng), CCT Otol (UK)
MBBS (Lond), MSB (UK), CBiol (Eur), MPhil (Lond),
MRCS Gen (Eng), DO-HNS (UK),
Consultant ENT, Thyroid & Nasal Plastic Surgeon
Head of ENT Department
Al Zahra Hospital, Sharjah
PO Box 3499, Sharjah, United Arab Emirates
Founder and Director of ENTTZAR, ENT CLUB & ENT ACADEMY
www.ricardopersaud.com

Dr Vishal Prasad

Lieutenant Commander
MBBS, MS, DNB (ENT) MRCSEd (ENT)
Specialist ENT Surgeon
iCARE Clinics, Dubai
Lamcy Plaza | Al Qusais
United Arab Emirates

Dr Adnan Darr

BSc, MSc, MBChB, DOHNS, MRCS (ENT)
ENT Registrar
Walsall Manor Hospital
England, UK

FIRST EDITION 2016

AF698839

FastPrint Publishing

http://www.fast-print.net/bookshop

ENT Head and Neck Surgery
Extended Matching Items

A catalogue record for this book is available from the British Library

ISBN 978-178456-418-6

First published 2016 by
FASTPRINT PUBLISHING
Peterborough, England.

About Extended Matching Items

Extended Matching Items (EMIs) are constructed to test factual recall and higher order thinking, such as application and evaluation of knowledge. They are therefore more clinically orientated in comparison to the multiple true/false MCQ questions. The EMIs cover a wider area of the syllabus, and usually assess clinically relevant information. It also extends beyond the simple recall of factual material and may assess the ability to interpret data from clinical scenarios.

A well constructed EMQ has four components:

1. A theme
2. A list of options
3. A lead-in statement
4. A list of stems

All the options are possible answers, which are based around the theme and may cover a wide area of the syllabus. The large number of options recuces the chance of guessing. If an answer is not obvious, then it is usually worth making a note of the likely possibilities and then choose the most likely answer by process of elimination (the answer is there!). Your initial response or 'gut feeling' is usually correct, and continually altering the chosen answer is not likely to improve the mark.

Be aware of the time limitations. This is important since there is little to be gained by spending a disproportionate amount of time on one question if it results in failing to complete the paper. The average time to answer a question is around 25 seconds. So pace yourself appropriately and answer all the questions.

CONTENT

CHAPTER 1

Paper 1

EMI Questions (Q1-Q100)

For each stem, select one correct answer option.

Theme: Branchial anomalies

Options for Questions 1–5

A First branchial arch
B First branchial cleft
C First branchial pouch
D Second branchial arch
E Second branchial cleft
F Second branchial pouch
G Third branchial arch
H Third branchial cleft
I Third branchial pouch
J Fourth branchial arch
K Fourth branchial cleft
L Fourth branchial pouch
M Sixth branchial arch
N Sixth branchial cleft

For each of the following cases, select the single most likely branchial apparatus responsible for the defect. Each option may be used once, more than once or not at all.

1. A 4-year-old girl presents with a discharge above the left tragus. Examination reveals a pre-auricular sinus.
2. A 7-year-old boy presents bilateral hearing loss. Examination reveals down slanting palpebral fissures, microtia, ear canal atresias and bilateral conductive hearing loss.
3. A 6-month-old boy presents with mild stridor. Investigations reveal laryngeal chondromalacia and double aortic arches.
4. A 2-year-old girl presents with discharge from a congenital opening anterior to the sternomastoid muscle. She is also partially deaf.
5. A 3-year-old boy presents with recurrent abscesses and inflammation which mimics acute suppurative thyroiditis.

Theme: Cause of epistaxis

Options for Questions 6–8

A Allergic rhinitis
B Drug induced
C Foreign body
D Iatrogenic
E Idiopathic
F Juvenile angio fibroma
G Malignant disease
H Osler-Weber-Rendu disease
I Pyogenic granuloma
J Rhinolith

K Sarcoidosis
L Substance abuse
M Trauma
N Wegener's granuloma

For each of the following cases, select the single most likely cause of epistaxis. Each option may be used once, more than once or not at all.

6. A 38-year-old woman presents with a long history of epistaxis. Anterior rhinoscopy reveals several red spots on the septal mucosa, also present on her lips and face.

7. A 2-year-old boy presents with a blood-stained, foul smelling mucopurulent discharge from one nostril. Examination reveals an inflamed nasal mucosa.

8. A 14-year-old girl presents with epistaxis. Anterior rhinoscopy reveals a smooth swollen red mass with contact bleeding.

Theme: Lymphatic drainage of the head and neck

Options for Questions 9–10

A Anterior cervical nodes
B Internal jugular nodes
C Jugulo-digastric nodes
D Jugulo-omohyoid nodes
E Occipital nodes
F Parotid nodes
G Post auricular nodes
H Posterior cervical nodes

I Posterior superficial cervical nodes
J Preauricular nodes
K Sublingual nodes
L Submandibular nodes
M Submental nodes
N Supraclavicular nodes

For each of the following statements regarding drainage of lymph, select the single most relevant node. Each option may be used once, more than once or not at all.

9. The palatine tonsils and lateral oropharyngeal wall drain into these nodes.

10. Lymphatic drainage from the tongue into these nodes prior to entering the jugular trunk.

Theme: Facial nerve palsy

Options for Questions 11–13

A Adenoid cystic carcinoma
B Bell's palsy
C Cerebello-pontine angle tumour
D Guillain-Barré
E Heerfordt
F Lyme disease
G Mononeuritis multiplex
H Multiple sclerosis
I Myasthenia gravis
J Ramsay Hunt
K Sarcoidosis
L Stroke

M Temporal bone fracture

For each of the following cases, select the single most likely diagnosis. Each option may be used once, more than once or not at all.

11. A 75-year-old man presents with a unilateral facial nerve weakness, associated with ipsilateral ear pain. Examination reveals vesicles in the painful ear.

12. A 32-year-old man was seen in ITU for tracheostomy decannulation. He was previously intubated because of generalised weakness and respiratory distress. He was noted to have bilateral facial nerve palsies. Six weeks prior to his admission he had a flu-like illness.

13. A 32-year-old woman presents with facial nerve palsy and joint pains. She had recently been on a walking holiday in Canada where she developed a flu-like illness associated with a rash.

Theme: Neck masses

Options for Questions 14–16

A Anaplastic thyroid cancer
B Branchial cyst
C Cystic hygroma
D Dermoid cyst
E Medullary thyroid carcinoma
F Papillary thyroid carcinoma
G Pilomatrixoma
H Teratoma
I Thyroglossal cyst

For each of the following cases, select the single most likely diagnosis. Each option may be used once, more than once or not at all.

14. A newborn baby boy is found to have a large swelling in the anterior neck. It extends retrosternally, causing compression and deviation of the trachea, with airway compromise requiring immediate intubation and ventilation. An urgent ultrasound scan and FNA reveals a heterogeneous mass, which contains a mixture of undifferentiated and differentiated cells.

15. A 47-year-old man presents with a 5 x 4 cm neck mass below the level of the hyoid bone. The lump first appeared following trauma to the neck during a rugby match. He was reassured by a casualty senior house officer that it would subside with time, as it was most likely to be a haematoma. It persisted and became infected twice requiring antibiotics. On examination, it does not move on swallowing or on tongue protrusion. Ultrasound scanning reveals a cystic lesion.

16. A 12-year-old boy presents with a midline neck anomaly, which has a dimple and a hair protruding from it.

Theme: Local anaesthetic doses

Options for Questions 17–19

A Bupivacaine

B Cocaine

C Levobupivacaine
D Lignocaine
E Prilocaine
F Ropivacaine

For each of the following maximum safe doses, select the single most appropriate local anaesthesia. Each option may be used once, more than once or not at all.

17. The maximum safe dose is 2 mg/kg without adrenaline.

18. The maximum safe dose is 3 mg/kg without adrenaline.

19. The maximum safe dose is 1.5 mg/kg, and duration of action is 30–60 min.

Theme: Headache

Options for Questions 20–23

A Benign (idiopathic) intracranial hypertension
B Cerebral abscess
C Cerebrovascular accident
D Cervical Spondylosis
E Cluster headache
F Giant cell arteritis
G Intracerebral haemorrhage
H Meningitis
I Migraine
J Psychogenic headache
K Space occupying lesion (e.g. brain tumour)
L Subarachnoid haemorrhage

M Temporomandibular joint (TMJ) dysfunction
N Tension (myofascial) headache

For each of the following cases, select the single most likely diagnosis. Each option may be used once, more than once or not at all.

20. A 24-year-old woman presents with a four-month history of severe, episodic throbbing left sided headaches associated tingling in her left hand. Prior to each episode, she feels unwell and her appetite subsides, especially chocolate, which she addicted to. She also describes flashing lights in her left visual field prior to the onset of the 'unbearable' headache. Her headache sometimes last for 72 hours. She describes being asymptomatic between attacks.

21. A 30-year-old man presents with a three-month history of severe, stabbing right sided headaches centred around the orbit, radiating to the cheek and jaw. The pain wakes him up from his sleep around 2 am every night, and he noticed his right eyes waters profusely. He seeks relief with paracetamol and pacing up and down. The headache lasts 40–60 minutes. The headache is not associated with any warning symptoms, visual disturbances or vomiting, but nasal congestion is present.

22. A 34-year-old woman presents to clinic with a three-month history of headache. It tends to occur when she is supine and is worse in the mornings. The headache is exacerbated by coughing, straining and bending over. She also complains of several episodes

of transient blurring of vision. Examination reveals an obese female with mild bilateral papilloedema. She has no other neurological signs.

23. A 72-year-old woman presents with a constant, throbbing generalised headache that has been increasing in intensity over a four-week period. She also notices pain on chewing. Examination reveals low grade pyrexia and a tender scalp, as well as decreased visual acuity in her right eye. ESR is elevated, but her CRP and temporal artery biopsy are reported as normal.

Theme: Skull base anatomy

Options for Questions 24–28

A Foramen Magnum
B Foramen Ovale
C Foramen Rotundum
D Foramen Spinosum
E Infratemporal fossa
F Jugular foramen
G Meckel's cave
H Optic canal
I Petrotympanic fissure
J Stylomastoid foramen

For each of the following anatomical statements, select the single most relevant associated structure. Each option may be used once, more than once or not at all.

24. Maxillary nerve passes through this opening to exit the cranial vault.

25. Permits entry of the middle meningeal artery to the cranium.

26. Houses the trigeminal ganglion.

27. The entry port of the spinal division of the accessory nerve into the cranium.

28. The exit port of the spinal division of the accessory nerve out of the cranium.

Theme: Sinonasal tumours

Options for Questions 29–33

A Adenocarcinoma
B Adenoid cystic carcinoma
C Angiofibroma
D Benign nasal polyps
E Cylindrical cell papillomas
F Fungiform papilloma
G Inverted papilloma
H Lymphoma
I Malignant melanoma
J Mucoepidermoid carcinoma
K Olfactory neuroblastoma
L Rhabdomyosarcoma
M Schneiderian papillomas
N Squamous cell carcinoma

For each of the following cases, select the single most likely diagnosis. Each option may be used once, more than once or not at all.

29. A 60-year-old male worker presents with blood stained nasal discharge. He works in a nickel factory.

30. A 49-year-old male carpenter presents with a blood stained nasal discharge.

31. A 40-year-old man presents with a warty lesion on the nasal septum, but no nasal discharge.

32. A 14-year-old boy presents with recurrent epistaxis. Examination reveals a unilateral nasal mass.

33. A 14-year-old boy presents with unilateral nasal obstruction. A CT scan reveals a unilateral homogenous maxillary mass, with destruction of the adjacent bone.

Theme: Viruses

Options for Questions 34–38

A Adenovirus
B Astrovirus
C Coxsackie virus
D Cytomegalovirus
E Epstein–Barr virus
F Hepatitis C virus
G Herpes simplex virus
H Herpes zoster virus
I Human papilloma virus

J Papovavirus
K Parainfluenza virus
L Paramyxovirus
M Parvovirus
N Rotavirus

For each of the following conditions, select the single most likely causative virus. Each option may be used once, more than once or not at all.

34. Subacute sclerosing panencephalitis.

35. Croup.

36. Infectious mononucleosis.

37. Laryngeal papillomatosis.

38. Aseptic meningitis.

Theme: Management of sleep disordered breathing in adults

Options for Questions 39–40

A Adenotonsillectomy
B Alcohol avoidance
C Continuous positive airway pressure (CPAP)
D Diathermy assisted uvuloplasty
E Exercise
F Laser-assisted uvuloplasty
G Mandibular advancement splint
H Oxygen therapy
I Pharyngeal wall surgery
J Sleeping tablet avoidance

K Somnoplasty
L Tongue base reduction
M Tracheostomy
N Weight loss

For each of the following cases, select the single most appropriate management option. Each option may be used once, more than once or not at all.

39. A 49-year-old male taxi driver presents complaining of snoring. He has had road traffic accidents, and suffers from claustrophobia. His body mass index is normal. A sleep study confirms moderate obstructive sleep apnoea.

40. A 49-year-old male obese patient presents complaining of snoring. His wife reports that he stops breathing several times each night, for over 10 sec. His sleep study reveals severe obstructive sleep apnoea with an AHI of 38.

Theme: ENT Eponyms

Options for Questions 41–44:

A Aquino's sign
B Bezold's sign
C Boyce
D Brown
E Bryce
F Citelle
G Furstenberg
H Gradenigo's syndrome

I Hennebert
J Hitselberger's sign
K Holman–Miller
L Schwartze's sign
M Semon's law
N Tullio phenomenon

For each of the following cases, select the single most likely eponymous name. Each option may be used once, more than once or not at all.

41. A 67-year-old woman presents with hearing loss on the left, and a decreased sensation along the floor of the ear canal and conchal bowl.

42. A 27-year-old woman presents with deafness following her pregnancy. Otoscopy reveals a pink tinge behind the tympanic membrane.

43. A 52-year-old man present with hearing loss and dizziness when he hears a loud noise such as his alarm clock.

44. A 4-year-old male child presents with a right discharging ear, fever and new onset squint in his right eye.

Theme: Tracheostomy tubes

Options for Questions 45–47

A Adjustable flange
B Cuffed fenestrated
C Cuffed non-fenestrated

D Silver negus single lumen
E Uncuffed fenestrated
F Uncuffed non-fenestrated

For each of the following cases, select the single most appropriate tracheostomy tube. Each option may be used once, more than once or not at all.

45. A 60-year-old man presents with 4-day-old tracheostomy tube in situ. He now requires upper airway airflow in order for him to speak.

46. A 25-year-old woman presents with airway obstruction secondary to laryngeal trauma sustained in a RTA. She requires a surgical tracheostomy to protect her airway.

47. A 50-year-old woman presents with severe septicaemia following abdominal surgery. Her BMI is 35, and she requires a tracheostomy for ventilation. The surgeon notes an increased pre-tracheal space due to excessive amount of adipose tissue.

Theme: Drug calculations

Options for Questions 48–51:

A 5 μg
B 10 μg
C 12 μg
D 120 μg
E 12.5 μg
F 125 μg
G 50 μg

H 500 μg
I 5 mg
J 10 mg
K 100 mg
L 200 mg
M 250 mg
N 225 mg

For each of the following solutions, calculate the single most likely amount of drug present. Each option may be used once, more than once or not at all.

48. The amount of cocaine present in 5 mL of Moffett's solution containing 2 mL of 10% cocaine.

49. The amount of adrenaline contained in 1 mL of 1:200,000 adrenaline solution.

50. The amount of adrenaline contained in 1 mL of 1:80,000 adrenaline solution.

51. The amount of lidocaine present in 100 μL (i.e. 1 puff) of Co-phenylcaine, which contains 5% lidocaine.

Theme: Conditions affecting the oral cavity

Options for Questions 52–56:

A Aphthous ulcer
B Cheilitis glandularis
C Erythroplakia
D Geographic tongue
E Leukoplakia
F Lichen Planus

G Mucocoeles
H Necrotising sialometaplasia
I Rhomboid glossitis
J Sialosis
K Sjögren's
L Subacute necrotising sialadenitis
M Traumatic ulcer
N Xerostomia

For each of the following cases, select the single most likely diagnosis. Each option may be used once, more than once or not at all.

52. A 65-year-old man presents with dry mouth and dental caries. He has taken Omeprazole daily for the last 2 years.

53. A 45-year-old woman presents with bilateral painless parotid swellings. She has diabetes.

54. A 50-year-old woman presents with early morning joint pains, dry eyes and dry mouth.

55. A 29-year-old man presents with a single recurrent blue sessile swelling on the lower lip that ruptures to release viscid salty mucous.

56. A 65-year-old man presents with sudden onset of palatal mass that breaks down to produce, painless irregular ulcer complaining of pyrexia and malaise

Theme: Choice of hearing devices

Options for Questions 57–60:

A Body-worn hearing aid
B Bone anchored hearing aid
C Bone conduction hearing aid
D Cochlear implant
E Implanted middle ear hearing aid
F In-the-canal (ITC) hearing aid
G In-the-ear (ITE) hearing aid
H No device
I Postaural hearing aid (unvented)
J Spectacle CROS hearing aid
K Vented behind-the-ear (BTE) hearing aid

For each of the following cases, select the single most appropriate initial hearing device. Each option may be used once, more than once or not at all.

57. A 25-year-old male professional surfer presents with recurrent otitis externa and moderate conductive hearing loss. Examination reveals bilateral sessile masses adjacent to the tympanic membrane in the external auditory canal.

58. A 35-year-old male company director complains of difficulty hearing in the presence of background noises. His pure tone audiometry reveals moderate hearing loss at 250 Hz but the thresholds at the other frequencies are all less than 20 dB HL.

59. A 70-year-old arthritic man from a nursing home complains of hearing loss. His pure tone audiograms reveal bilateral severe sensorineural hearing loss.

60. A 19-year-old female student presents with single-sided sensorineural deafness following as road traffic accident. She is also short sighted and severely needle phobic.

Theme: Dynamic airway test

Options for Questions 61–63:

A Acoustic rhinometry
B Manometric rhinometry
C Nasal expiratory peak flow
D Nasal inspiratory peak flow
E Peak flow
F Rhinomanometry
G Rhinostereometry
H Spatula misting
I Spirometry

For each of the following assessments, select the single most appropriate test. Each option may be used once, more than once or not at all.

61. To assess nasal respiration.

62. To assess pulmonary function in asthmatic patients.

63. To assess volume at different distances into the nose.

Theme: TNM STAGING

Options for Questions 64–65

A T1N0M0
B T1N1M0

C T1N1aM0
D T1N1bM0
E T2N0M0
F T2N1M0
G T3N0M0
H T3N1M0
I T4N0M0
J T4N1M0

For each of the following cases, select the single most appropriate TNM stage. Each option may be used once, more than once or not at all.

64. A 45-year-old man presents with a four-month history of persistent ear ache and some discomfort swallowing, but no weight loss. He has consumed 10 units of alcohol daily for 5 years. Examination reveals a 3 cm cancerous ulcer in the left piriform fossa, extending from the medial wall to the lateral wall. Vocal folds were mobile and symmetrical. Neck examination was normal with no palpable lymph nodes.

65. A 59-year-old Asian man presents with a history of nasal obstruction and epistaxis. CT scanning shows a mass in the left ethmoid sinus invading the orbit but not the extending intracranially. There are no neck nodes.

Theme: Genetic syndromes in ENT practice

Options for Questions 66–68

A	Alport
B	Alstrom
C	Beckwith–Wiedemann
D	Branchiootorenal
E	CHARGE
F	Goldenhar
G	Jervell–Lange-Neilsen
H	Pendred
I	Solitary median maxillary central incisor
J	Sticklers
K	Treacher–Collins
L	Turners
M	Velocardiofacial
N	Waardenburg

For each of the following cases, select the single most likely syndrome. Each option may be used once, more than once or not at all.

66. A 4-year-old boy presents with hearing loss. Examination reveals mandibular and midfacial hypoplasia along with down slanting palpabre fissures.

67. A 10-year-old boy presents with a pre-auricular sinus and mucoid discharge from a small pit in his neck. He is under the care of the renal physician. Investigations reveal bilaterally sensorineural deafness.

68. A 10-month-old girl presents with difficulty breathing. On examination, she is noted to be obese with significant macroglossia.

Theme: Nystagmus

Options for Questions 69–73

- A Bidirectional
- B Downbeat
- C Horizontal to the left
- D Horizontal to the right
- E No nystagmus
- F Pendular
- G Rotatory geotropic to the left
- H Rotatory geotropic to the right
- I Upbeat
- J Vertical

For each of the following cases, select the single most likely type of nystagmus to be present. Each option may be used once, more than once or not at all.

69. A 62-year-old male sailor is noted to have a fistula in the lateral semicircular canal during right tympanomastoid surgery. It is associated with gushing of clear fluid, which is impossible to control with a temporalis fascia graft only. Control of fluid flow is achieved with bone wax applied to the defect. The patient wakes up feeling extremely dizzy. A Weber tuning fork test goes to the left suggesting a right dead ear.

70. A 42-year-old male office worker is noted to have a fistula of the lateral semicircular canal during right tympanomastoid surgery. There is no fluid leak, and the defect is filled with bone wax. The patient wakes up feeling dizzy. A Weber tuning fork test went to the right.

71. A 35-year-old woman is found to have nystagmus when her head is turned to the right during a Hallpike manoeuvre.

72. A 48-year-old man presents with congenital blindness and nystagmus.

73. A 10-year-old boy presents with an Arnold Chiari Malformation and is noted to have nystagmus.

Theme: Hearing Loss

Options for Questions 74–75:

A Benign intracranial hypertension
B Cochlear hydrops
C Cochlear otosclerosis
D Cogan's syndrome
E Enlarged vestibular aqueduct syndrome
F Heredito-degenerative disease of the cochlea
G Inner ear conductive presbyacusis
H Mondini inner ear deformity
I Neural presbyacusis
J Refsum's syndrome
K Tympanosclerosis
L Strial presbyacusis

M Syphilitic ear
N Usher's syndrome

For each of the following cases, select the single most appropriate diagnosis from the above list. Each option may be used once, more than once or not at all.

74. A 14-year-old boy presents with conductive hearing loss, with significant whitish discolouration of the tympanic membrane surrounding a healed monomeric segment of the drum. The patient previously had two sets of grommets.

75. A 14-year-old boy presents with progressive sensorineural hearing loss, which suddenly worsens following head trauma whilst playing rugby.

Theme: Aetiopathogenesis of cholesteatoma

Options for Questions 76–80

A Acquired inclusion theory
B Amniotic fluid contamination theory
C Basal hyperplasia theory
D Embryonic germ cell distribution theory
E Epidermoid formation theory
F Epithelial migration theory
G Iatrogenic or post-traumatic theory
H Migration theory
I Retraction pocket theory
J Squamous metaplasia theory

For each of the following statements pertaining to the pathogenesis of cholesteatoma, select the single most likely theory. Each option may be used once, more than once or not at all.

76. Involves the persistence of a small nest of stratified squamous epithelial cells.

77. Involves mainly the pars flaccida and negative middle ear pressure.

78. Involves rete ridges of the basement membrane.

79. Involves the epithelium around the margin of a tympanic membrane perforation.

80. Involves the transformation of cuboidal epithelial tissue to stratified squamous keratinising tissue.

Theme: Glasgow Coma Score (GCS)

Options for Questions 81–83:

A 3
B 4
C 5
D 6
E 7
F 8
G 9
H 10
I 11
J 12
K 13
L 14
M 15

For each of the following cases, select the single most likely GCS. Each option may be used once, more than once or not at all.

81. A 17-year-old man is involved in a road traffic accident. He has no response to commands, and only extends his arm to pain. His eyes remain closed.

82. A 78-year-old female patient sits up in bed, with eyes wide open, answers questions but is not making sense.

83. A 25-year-old woman presents following an assault, opens her eyes spontaneously and is able to localise painful stimuli, but mumbles inappropriate words.

Theme: Soft tissue lesions on the nose

Options for Questions 84–86:

A Basal cell carcinoma
B Haemangioma
C Melanoma
D Nasal dermoid
E Nasal glioma
F Nasoalveolar cyst
G Papilloma
H Rhinophyma
I Squamous cell carcinoma

For each of the following cases, select the single most appropriate diagnosis. Each option may be used once, more than once or not at all.

84. A 58-year-old man presents with difficulty breathing through his nose because of a long standing bulbous lesion on his nose. This has become ruddy and vascular in appearance.

85. A 5-year-old boy presents with a swelling near the glabella, which has been present since birth. It has a pit and is firm to palpation.

86. A 63-year-old woman presents with pearly lesion, with an ulcerated centre on her nose. She spends a lot of time in the Caribbean.

Theme: Imaging

Options for Questions 87–91:

A CT scan with contrast
B CT scan without contrast
C FDG PET CT
D Gadolinium enhanced MRI scan
E MRI non echo planar diffusion weighted
F MRI STIR sequence
G MRI T1 images
H MRI T2 images
I Ultrasound
J X -ray

For each of the following cases, select the single most appropriate imaging modality. Each option may be used once, more than once or not at all.

87. A 39-year-old man presents with a parotid gland mass. The surgeon would like to know if the lesion extends to the deep lobe of the parotid gland.

88. A 65-year-old woman presents with asymmetrical sensory neural hearing loss without tinnitus.

89. A 15-year-old girl who had combined approach tympanoplasty 12 months ago for cholesteatoma. The surgeon would like to know if the disease has recurred.

90. A 60-year-old man presents with metastatic neck disease of unknown primary. MRI neck was reported as normal.

91. A 55-year-old woman presents with spontaneous CSF rhinorrhoea. Her BMI is 38.

Theme: Analgesia

Options for Questions 92–94:

A Aspirin
B Codeine
C Diclofenac
D Benzydamine hydrochloride
E Morphine
F Oxybutynin
G Paracetamol
H Tramadol

For each of the following pharmacological statements, select the single most relevant associated drug. Each option may be used once, more than once or not at all.

92. This drug is a weak opioid and a pro-drug. It possesses weak agonist actions at the μ-opioid receptor, releases serotonin and inhibits the reuptake of norepinephrine.

93. This drug is an anti-pyretic agent that is hepatotoxic in overdose.

94. This drug is associated with Reye's syndrome in children.

Theme: Fine Needle Aspiration Cytology (FNAC) of the thyroid gland

Options for Questions 95–96:

A Thy1
B Thy2
C Thy3
D Thy4
E Thy5

For each of the following cases, select the single most appropriate Thy stage. Each option may be used once, more than once or not at all.

95. A 38-year-old woman presents with a thyroid swelling. Fine needle aspiration cytology suggests a follicular thyroid lesion.

96. A 17-year-old man presents with a thyroid lesion. Fine needle aspiration cytology suggests a non-neoplastic result.

Theme: Statistical testings

Options for Questions 97–100:

A Chi-squared (χ2) test
B Fisher's exact-test
C Friedman test
D F-test
E Kruskal–Wallis test
F Mann–Whitney U test
G McNemar
H One sample (paired) Student's t-test
I One-way analysis of variance (ANOVA)
J Pearson's correlation coefficient
K Spearman's rank correlation coefficient
L Two sample (unpaired) Student's t-test
M Two-way analysis of variance (ANOVA)
N Wilcoxon matched pairs test

For each of the following data sets, select the single most suitable statistical test. Each option may be used once, more than once or not at all.

97. Visual analogue scale responses of a group of subjects (n = 16), who were asked to report their perceived contentment on two consecutive days.

98. The variation of weight over a period of 3 months, in 600 obese subjects on a calorie controlled weight reducing diet.

99. Comparing average blood pressures between a group of men and women.

100. The number of GP consultations in the first 10 years of life was obtained for a group of 200 children. Their parents were asked to complete a parenting skills questionnaire, from which a skills score (an integer value ranging from 0–25) was determined. The aim was to assess whether low parenting skills are related to a higher number of GP consultations.

Answer Keys to Chapter 1 EMIs

1	A	First branchial arch. ➢ Avoid temptation to put first branchial cleft, as the answer (pre-auricular sinuses arise from abnormal development of the otic hillocks of His, derived from the first and second branchial arches).
2	A	First branchial arch. ➢ The signs are consistent with Treacher–collins syndrome (one of the first arch syndromes, i.e., congenital malformations of the face due to failure of development of first arch structures).
3	J	Fourth branchial arch. ➢ Anomalies of the fourth branchial arch are uncommon entities and include asymmetric or stenotic larynx, chondromalacia and double aortic arch.
4	E	Second branchial cleft. ➢ Relatively common and result from failure to obliterate the second cleft by the inferior extension of the second arch. ➢ This results in an opening onto the skin in the anterior neck, usually at the anterior border of sternomastoid in

		the lower third of the neck.
5	I	Third branchial pouch. ➢ Abnormality can result in undescended or accessory parathyroid glands, thymic cysts or sinus tracts from the piriform fossa to the region of the thyroid gland. ➢ Diagnosis - Contrast swallow X-ray or by direct pharyngoscopy, where the sinus opening can be seen. ➢ Treatment is surgical excision of the tract or by endoscopic cautery of the tract seen in the piriform fossa.
6	H	Osler–Weber–Rendu. ➢ Autosomal dominant disorder, also known as hereditary familial telangiectasia (HHT). Due to a defect in the TGF-β signaling pathway, which results in deficient contractile connective tissue surrounding endovascular endothelium. ➢ An acute bleed should be managed with kaltostat soaked in adrenaline rather than merocel packs, which cause excessive trauma. Other form of therapy includes oestrogen, progesterone, KTP laser, septodermoplasty and Youngs procedure.

7	C	Foreign body. ➢ They are found most commonly amongst 2–3-year-old toddlers and are usually impacted between the septum and inferior turbinate. ➢ Any foul-smelling unilateral nasal discharge in a child, with excoriation of the vestibular skin, must be assumed to be due to a foreign body until proven otherwise.
8	I	Pyogenic granuloma. ➢ Typically pyogenic granulomas can grow rapidly and will often bleed profusely with little or no trauma. ➢ They may be confused with a haemangioma at first, but pyogenic granulomas grow rapidly and never involute like a haemangioma. ➢ Examination under anaesthesia, followed by surgical excision is usually curative. It is actually a capillary haemangioma of lobular subtype, which is why it is prone to bleeding. The granuloma is not truly pyogenic as the origin is traumatic and not infectious.
9	C	Jugulo-digastric nodes ➢ The jugulodigastric node is part of the deep lateral cervical group of nodes. It lies behind the posterior belly of the

		digastric muscle and anterior to the internal jugular vein. ➢ The jugulodigastric node receives lymphatic drainage from the lateral oropharyngeal wall, palatine tonsil and tongue. It is also called subdigastric node.
10	D	Jugulo-omohyoid nodes ➢ The jugulo-omohyoid node lies above the intermediate tendon of omohyoid muscle, and anterior to the internal jugular vein. It receives lymphatic drainage from the submental, submandibular, and deep anterior cervical nodes. ➢ Lymph drainage from the tongue reaches this node on both sides of the neck before entering the jugular trunks, and so a minimum level I–III neck dissection is required with tongue cancers (supra-omohyoid neck dissection).
11	J	Ramsay Hunt Syndrome. ➢ This syndrome consists of a very painful, erythematous, vesicular rash and a seventh cranial nerve lower motor neuron palsy, both of which are due to re-activation of the chicken pox virus, varicella zoster. ➢ Herpes zoster oticus is sometimes

		used to refer to Ramsay Hunt syndrome or when the ear alone is affected. Vesicles may therefore present in the distribution of the facial nerve.
12	D	Guillain–Barré Syndrome. ➢ This condition represents an acute polyneuropathy, which is thought to be an autoimmune cellular response directed against the myelin sheath of peripheral nerves. Patients often develop ascending sensory and motor symptoms several weeks after the onset of an infection. ➢ Most patients recover spontaneously, but steroids are still given together with supportive care. Severe cases may require ventilatory support due to involvement of the respiratory muscles. Plasma exchange and intravenous human immunoglobulin may also be necessary.
13	F	Lyme disease ➢ Lyme disease is zoonosis caused by a tick borne spirochaetal infection (*Borrelia burgdorferi)* carried on deer. Lyme's disease is endemic in certain parts of North America and Europe. ➢ Diagnosis of Lyme disease involves MRI and serological testing for

		Borrelia antibodies in blood and CSF (IgG and IgM). Sensorineural hearing loss may be the only symptom of neuro borreliosis.
14	H	Teratoma ➢ Encapsulated tumour with tissue or organ components resembling normal derivatives of all three germ layers. All tumours of this class are the result of abnormal development of pluripotent cells, germ cells and embryonal cells. ➢ Teratomas of embryonic origin are congenital; teratomas of germ cell origin may or may not be congenital. ➢ Teratomas commonly are classified using the Gonzalez–Crussi grading system: 0 or mature (benign); 1 or immature, probably benign; 2 or immature, possibly malignant (cancerous); and 3 or frankly malignant. Teratomas rarely become malignant.
15	I	Thyroglossal cyst ➢ This is an interesting case of a dormant thyroglossal duct cyst becoming evident after trauma, and emphasises the general principle that trauma often leads to presentation of pre-existing non-traumatic lesions. ➢ The thyroid gland remains connected

		to the foramen caecum by the thyroglossal duct, which eventually involutes and disappears. A thyroglossal cyst results from the persistence of the thyroglossal duct, or part of the duct and may appear at any point in the migratory pathway taken by the thyroid gland during it development, including the thyroid *per se*. ➢ In up to 20% of cases, thyroglossal cysts may be found lateral to the midline, most often on the left, probably because of the presence of the asymmetrical levator glandulae thyroidaea, which connects the thyroid to the hyoid bone. ➢ Classically, a thyroglossal cyst moves upwards on tongue protrusion.
16	D	Dermoid cyst ➢ It is a mature cystic teratoma containing hairs (sometimes very abundant) and other structures characteristic of normal skin and other tissues derived from the ectoderm. ➢ In the neck, dermoid cysts occur in the submental region, deep or superficial to mylohyoid membrane and may mimic a ranula.
17	A	Bupivacaine

		➢ Local anaesthetic drugs work by blocking sodium channels within the axon, causing a reversible block to conduction along nerve fibres. ➢ Bupivacaine has a long duration of action (240 minutes without adrenaline) and therefore useful for post-operative analgesia. Max dose is 2 mg/kg or 3 mg/kg with adrenaline. ➢ Bupivacaine with adrenaline is available as an injection of anhydrous bupivacaine hydrochloride 5 mg/mL (0.5%) with 1:200,000 (5 µg /mL) adrenaline. The trade name for bupivacaine is marcain and it comes in a clear plastic container as it is not light sensitive like cocaine
18	D	Lignocaine ➢ Lignocaine or lidocaine is an amide local anaesthetic. It acts on the sodium channels to cause a reversible conduction block along nerves. The addition of a vasoconstrictor speeds up the onset of action and prolongs the local anaesthetic effect. Plain lidocaine is expected to last 2 hours, however with the addition of adrenaline (epinephrine) this is extended up to 4 hours. ➢ The recommended safe dose of:

		Plain lidocaine is 3 mg/kg Lidocaine with adrenaline is 7 mg/kg. Adrenaline 4 µg/kg ➢ Lidocaine is available as an injectable liquid (0.5–2%), spray (4% or 10%) and ointments (2–5%). It is a mild vasodilator. Its duration of action is about 90 minutes with adrenaline. ➢ Lidocaine given intravenously affects central auditory pathways and the cochlea to produce short term relief of tinnitus but has cardiac side effects.
19	B	Cocaine ➢ In contrast to the other local anaesthetic, cocaine has vasoconstrictor properties and is rapidly effective on mucous membranes. Cocaine is an ester local anaesthetic (one way to distinguish an ester from an amide is that the former has only one 'i.' in the name whilst the latter has two). ➢ The max safe dose is 1.5 mg/kg, although some books recommend up to 3 mg/kg. Its duration of action is 30–60 min. ➢ Immediate management of cocaine overdose involves intravenous administration of diazepam to control

		agitation, as well as cooling measures for hyperthermia. Cocaine comes in either 5 or 10% solution. Cocaine paste is no longer used because of the potential risk of vCJD.
20	I	Migraine ➢ The headache is usually unilateral, but may be generalised, and often associated with nausea, vomiting and/or visual disturbances including flashing lights. ➢ Other symptoms may be present such as tingling in the face or ipsilateral limb. ➢ Animal studies suggest that the trigeminovascular system is the common pathway leading to migraine. ➢ The headache can be precipitated by numerous factors, such as psychological stress, endocrine changes (e.g. menstruation) and certain foods, especially those containing tyramine (e.g. chocolate and aged cheeses). ➢ Management involves avoidance of any recognised precipitating factors, and symptomatic relief with analgesia and anti-emetics. If these are inadequate, sumatriptan, a 5HT1 antagonist may be required, and in

		more severe cases prophylaxis with a beta blocker, pizotifen, or diltiazem. Other treatments include acupuncture, hypnosis, stress management and Botox injections.
21	E	Cluster headache. ➢ Occurs in clusters consisting of 1–8 attacks per day for one to four months. Each attack usually lasts for about 1 hour. The cluster of headaches is followed by a symptom-free period, which can be as long as 18 months. ➢ The headaches are often unilateral, severe and come on at the same time during the day and/or night. They are always associated with autonomic phenomena such as runny eyes, injected conjunctivae, rhinorrhoea, nasal congestion and transient Horner's syndrome (25% of cases). There are no associated warning symptoms such as those seen in migrainous headache. ➢ The male to female ratio is 7:1 and the age of onset is between 20–40 years. ➢ Ergotamine, subcutaneously or by inhaler, is the mainstay of treatment and it is given just before the predicted start of an attack.

		Sphenopalatine ganglion block with intranasal local anaesthetic is also effective.
22	A	Benign idiopathic intracranial hypertension. ➢ Most sufferers of this type of headache are obese females. The headache is typically worsened by temporary changes in CSF pressure such as in coughing, straining and bending forward. ➢ Unlike migraine, papilloedema is commonly present and results in transient visual disturbances. In contrast with other causes of raised intracranial pressure, cognitive defects and deterioration of conscious level are rare. ➢ Patients with benign intracranial hypertension may also present to the Otolaryngologist with spontaneous CSF rhinorrhoea, and pulsatile tinnitus. ➢ Treatment is with acetazolamide (Diamox), analgesics. Low dose of the antidepressant amitriptyline, or the anticonvulsant topiramate has shown some additional benefit for pain relief. ➢ Surgery may be required if medical treatment fails: optic nerve sheath decompression and fenestration and

		shunting. Obese patients may benefit from gastric bypass procedure, which has been shown to improve symptoms.
23	F	Giant cell arteritis. ➢ Chronic inflammatory condition associated with non-specific signs such as fever, malaise and weight loss. ➢ It is due to ischaemia caused by inflammatory infiltration with subsequent obliteration of the lumen of the large arteries of the scalp, face and eyes, resulting in headache, diplopia, transient blurring of vision or even blindness. The scalp overlying the temporal artery is often tender. Claudication of the jaw and tongue may occur during mastication. ➢ ESR but not CRP is usually grossly elevated. Temporal artery biopsy is the definitive investigation, but inflammatory involvement may be local, so is only positive in 70% of cases.
24	C	Foramen rotundum ➢ Lies in the greater wing of the sphenoid bone that connects the middle cranial fossa to the pterygopalatine fossa. The maxillary division of the trigeminal nerve exits

		through this foramina. ➢ The foramen rotundum evolves in shape throughout the fetal period, and also from birth to adolescence. It reaches a perfect ring-shaped structure in the fetus after the 4th fetal month. Generally, it is mostly oval-shaped in the fetal period, and round-shaped after birth. After birth, the rotundum is about 2.5 mm and in 15-to 17-year olds about 3 mm in length. The average diameter of the foramen rotundum in adults is approximately 3.55 mm.
25	D	Foramen spinosum ➢ Lies in the greater wing of the sphenoid bone in the middle cranial fossa. It allows passage of the middle meningeal vein and artery as well as meningeal branch of the mandibular nerve (V3). The foramen may be absent (in approx. 2% of the cases) and in such cases the middle meningeal artery enters the cranial cavity through the foramen ovale. ➢ The foramen spinosum and ovale may be continuous, and the foramen spinosum may be duplicated. The foramen spinosum is more or less incomplete in approx. 44% of the

		cases. Occasionally the foramen spinosum was small or altogether absent in 0.4% of cases. This is especially true when the middle meningeal artery arises from the ophthalmic artery (the foramen would be near to empty in that case). In rare cases, early division of the middle meningeal artery into a posterior and anterior division may result in a duplication of the foramen spinosum. ➢ In the newborn, the foramen spinosum is about 2.25 mm, and in the adults about 2.56 mm in length. The width of the foramen extends from 1.05 mm to about 2.1 mm in the adults. The average diameter of the foramen spinosum is 2.63 mm in the adult.
26	G	Meckel's Cave ➢ Meckel's cave is two layers of dura mater that is formed by the invagination of the tentorium cerebelli. The boundaries are: ➢ Superolaterally: The cerebellar tentorium (tentorium cerebelli) Superomedially: The lateral wall of the cavernous sinus Medially: The clivus Inferolaterally: The posterior petrous

		bone Content - The trigeminal ganglion. ➢ Meckel's cave may be involved either by extrinsic or intrinsic disease. ➢ Extrinsic lesions, usually bony metastasis, chordoma, or chondrosarcoma, destroy adjacent bone as they extend toward the Meckel's cave. Intrinsic lesions simply expand the Meckel's cave. When the tumour is large enough, the pressure exerted by it leads to erosion of the surrounding bone. Tumours can also extend away from the Meckel's cave with enlargement of the foramen ovale basis cranii, foramen rotundum, or the superior orbital fissure. ➢ Intrinsic lesions include primary tumors of the Meckel's cave as well as secondary neoplasms from perineural spread of local tumors, leptomeningeal, or hematogenous metastasis. Primary tumours of the Meckel's cavity include trigeminal schwannoma, meningioma, and epidermoid cyst.
27	A	Foramen magnum ➢ Foramen magnum is in the occipital bone in the posterior cranial fossa. ➢ The spinal part of the accessory nerve

		is the only cranial nerve to start its journey outside the skull. It enters through the foramen magnum. ➢ Other structures passing through - medulla oblongata, meninges, vertebral arteries, anterior and posterior spinal arteries, sympathetic plexus on the vertebral arteries, apical ligament of dens and tectorial membrane. ➢ It is the unpaired foramen posteriorly whilst the foramen caecum is the unpaired foramen anteriorly. The foramen caecum normally transmits an emissary vein.
28	F	Jugular foramen ➢ The spinal accessory travels in the floor of the cranium from the foramen magnum to the jugular foramen, where it exits to innervate sternocleidomastoid and trapezium. The cranial accessory rapidly joins the vagus, and is involved in innervation of palatopharyngeus and the three constrictors. ➢ The jugular foramen may be subdivided into three compartments, each with their own contents. The anterior compartment - inferior petrosal sinus, the intermediate – IX,

		X, XI CNs, the posterior - sigmoid sinus, which becomes the internal jugular vein, and some meningeal branches from the occipital and ascending pharyngeal arteries. ➢ An alternative imaging based classification exists, using the jugular spine, which is a bony ridge partially separating the jugular foramen, into two parts. The smaller, anteromedial, 'pars nervosa' compartment contains CN IX, Jacobson nerve (or the tympanic nerve, a branch of CN IX), and receives the venous return from inferior petrosal sinus. The larger, posterolateral, 'pars vascularis' compartment contains CN X, CN XI, Arnold's nerve (or the auricular branch of CN X involved in the Arnold's reflex, where external auditory meatus stimulation causes cough), jugular bulb, posterior meningeal artery (branch of vertebral artery), and meningeal branch of ascending pharyngeal artery.
29	N	Squamous cell carcinoma. ➢ The most common sinonasal malignant tumour. The maxillary sinus is the most common site of occurrence, followed by the nasal

		cavity and then the ethmoid sinus. ➢ Diagnosis is usually delayed because the symptoms of sinonasal squamous cell carcinoma resemble benign sinusitis, for example, unilateral nasal obstruction, minor epistaxis, nasal discharge and low grade infection. More advanced tumour may present with tooth pain, proptosis, trismus and headache when there is invasion of the palate, orbit, infratemporal fossa and anterior skull base, respectively. ➢ Squamous cell carcinoma and adenocarcinoma are associated with exposure to products found in furniture making, the leather industry, and the textile industry: Wood dust, nickel dust, Mustard gas, Isopropyl oil, Chromium, Dichlorodiethyl sulfide. Some viral infections can cause sinus cancer. The human papilloma virus (HPV) can produce a benign (non-cancerous) sinus tumor called inverted papilloma.
30	A	Adenocarcinoma. ➢ Associated with hardwood workers and is the second most common sinonasal malignancy. The most common site of origin is the ethmoid

		sinus. It tends to spread in the nasal cavity rather than through the cribriform plate. ➢ Adenocarcinoma starts in the gland cells (adenomatous cells) that are scattered around the surface tissues inside the nose and produce mucus. The number of adenocarcinomas appears to have increased in the last 20 years, probably because of better detection methods. ➢ Adenoid cystic cancers are rare cancers of gland tissue. They most often grow in the salivary glands but, much more rarely, can grow in the nose or nasal sinuses.
31	F	Fungiform papilloma. ➢ Three histologically distinct papillomas are present in the sinonasal cavity: fungiform, inverted and cylindric papillomas; collectively they are called Schneiderian papillomas. ➢ The fungiform varieties usually occur in males aged 40–70 years, and about 95% arise from the nasal septum. They have a warty or verrucous appearance, and therefore may be caused by human papilloma virus. They are unlikely to undergo

		malignant transformation. Treatment is by surgical excision, but recurrence may occur. ➢ Inverted papillomas tend to arise from the lateral nasal wall and may undergo malignant transformation in 9–13% of cases. Definitive treatment involves endoscopic medial maxillectomy. ➢ Cylindrical cell papillomas are relatively rare, and arise from the maxillary sinus. Macroscopically the lesions tend to be more friable than inverted papillomas. Histologically, they are covered with ciliated respiratory epithelium with cystic stroma containing mucus. Treatment is endoscopic removal.
32	C	Angiofibroma. ➢ Benign, but locally aggressive tumour arising form the posterolateral nasal wall adjacent to the pterygopalatine foramen. ➢ The typical presentation is in an adolescent male with recurrent nose bleeds. Any female with this condition needs to undergo chromosomal analysis. ➢ The lesion should never be biopsied. Diagnosis is made on history,

		examination and imaging. The tumour typically causes anterior bowing of the ipsilateral posterior maxillary wall (pathognomonic Holman–Miller sign). ➢ Post surgical recurrence may be prevented by drilling out the vidian canal and basisphenoid region at the time of primary surgery. ➢ Medical treatment, such as diethylstilbestrol, to make the lesion less vascular may be given before surgery. ➢ Embolisation of the feeding vessels (most often ascending pharyngeal artery) also reduces intra-operative blood loss. ➢ Lesions extending into the cranial cavity or whose tumors can't be safely reached by surgery, may be treated with radiotherapy. Radiation therapy helps in case where recurrence is the main problem.
33	L	Rhabdomyosarcoma. ➢ Rare cancer of connective tissue type, in which the cancer cells arise from skeletal muscle progenitors. This tumour tends to occur in the head and neck region of children under 15-years-old. ➢ The two most common types are

embryonal rhabdomyosarcoma and alveolar rhabdomyosarcoma. Soft tissue sarcomas make up about 3% of childhood cancers.

- The diagnosis of rhabdomyosarcoma is made using immunohistochemical stain, and depends on recognition of differentiation toward skeletal muscle cells.
- Early manifestation can be misdiagnosed as a pseudotumor, which is unresponsive to steroid treatment. Prognosis and clinical behavior of the tumour is dependent on histologic subtype.
- Multiple classification systems have been proposed for subclassifying these tumors. The most recent classification system, the 'International Classification of Rhabdomyosarcoma', was created by the Intergroup Rhabdomyosarcoma Study.
- Treatment for rhabdomyosarcoma consists of chemotherapy, radiation therapy and occasionally surgery, which may be difficult or impossible because of the location of the tumour. If there is no evidence of metastasis, surgery combined with chemotherapy

		and radiation offers the best prognosis.
34	L	Paramyxovirus ➢ Subacute sclerosing panencephalitis is caused by persistent infection with the defective paramyxovirus virus, following primary measles infection several years previously. ➢ It is a severe progressive neurological condition that presents with personality changes and intellectual impairment, followed by convulsions, myoclonic movements, coma and death. ➢ Paramyxoviruses cause a number of important human diseases, including mumps, measles, and respiratory syncytial virus (RSV), which is the major cause of bronchiolitis and pneumonia in infants and children. ➢ Paramyxoviruses are also responsible for a range of diseases in other animal species, for example canine distemper virus (dogs), phocine distemper virus (seals), cetacean morbillivirus (dolphins and porpoises) Newcastle disease virus (birds), and rinderpest virus (cattle). Some paramyxoviruses such as the henipaviruses are zoonotic pathogens, but they are capable of

		infecting humans.
35	K	Parainfluenza virus. ➢ Croup or acute laryngotracheobronchitis is most commonly associated with parainfluenza RNA virus type 1. ➢ The symptoms of this condition include hoarseness, barking cough and stridor. The condition is mainly seen in infants and young children. ➢ Parainfluenza virus is also associated with bronchiolitis and pneumonia in children and the common cold in adults. Repeated infection throughout the life of the host is not uncommon. ➢ In immunosuppressed people, such as transplant patients, parainfluenza virus infections can cause severe pneumonia, which can be fatal. ➢ Parainfluenza viruses last only a few hours in the environment and are inactivated by soap and water, although no vaccines currently exist.
36	E	Epstein Barr virus. ➢ Infectious mononucleosis is a multisystem disease caused by Epstein Barr virus, also called human herpesvirus 4 (HHV-4), which is a DNA virus that belongs to the herpes virus family.

		➢ It is best known as the cause of infectious mononucleosis. It is also associated with particular forms of cancer, particularly Hodgkin's lymphoma, Burkitt's lymphoma, nasopharyngeal carcinoma, and central nervous system lymphomas associated with HIV. ➢ Infection with the virus is associated with a higher risk of certain autoimmune diseases, especially dermatomyositis systemic lupus erythematosus, rheumatoid arthritis, Sjögren's syndrome, and multiple sclerosis. Infants become susceptible to EBV as soon as maternal antibody protection disappears.
37	I	Human papilloma virus. ➢ All papillomas or warts are caused by human papilloma virus (HPV), a DNA virus belonging to the papovavirus family. Like all papillomaviruses, HPVs establish productive infections only in keratinocytes of the skin or mucous membranes. ➢ Some types can cause warts (verrucae), while others can lead to cancers of the cervix, vulva, vagina, and anus or cancers of the anus and penis. It can also cause cancers of the

		head and neck (tongue, tonsils and throat). ➢ HPV types 6 and 11 can cause a rare condition known as recurrent respiratory papillomatosis, in which warts form on the larynx or other areas of the respiratory tract. ➢ Two vaccines are available to prevent infection by some HPV types: Gardasil and Cervarix. Both protect against initial infection with HPV types 16 and 18, which cause most of the HPV associated cancer cases. Gardasil also protects against HPV types 6 and 11, which cause 90% of genital warts.
38	C	Coxsackie virus. ➢ Aseptic meningitis is usually due to viruses of the enterovirus group, of which Coxsackie virus is a member. Other enteroviruses that cause aseptic meningitis include echovirus and poliovirus. ➢ Coxsackieviruses are divided into group A and group B viruses. At least twenty-three serotypes (1–22, 24) of group A and six serotypes (1–6) of group B are recognized. Generally, group A coxsackieviruses tend to infect the skin and mucous membranes, causing herpangina,

		acute hemorrhagic conjunctivitis, and hand, foot and mouth (HFM) disease. ➢ Both group A and group B coxsackieviruses can cause nonspecific febrile illnesses, rashes, upper respiratory tract disease, and aseptic meningitis. ➢ Group B coxsackieviruses tend to infect the heart, pleura, pancreas, and liver, causing pleurodynia, myocarditis, pericarditis, and hepatitis (inflammation of the liver not related to the hepatotropic viruses). ➢ Insulin-dependent diabetes (IDDM) has recently been associated with recent enteroviral infection, particularly coxsackievirus B pancreatitis. Sjögren's syndrome is also being studied in connection with coxsackievirus.
39	G	Mandibular advancement splint. ➢ This is worth trying first in this patient as he is claustrophobic and therefore unlikely to tolerate CPAP. ➢ The splint is a tailored-made dental device that helps to keep the jaw forward and aids upper airway muscle tone during sleep. ➢ Obstructive sleep apnoea may be due to loss of upper airway/pharyngeal

		muscle tone during rapid eye movement sleep. ➢ First line management is aimed a life style changes such as less alcohol, weight loss and exercise. Tracheostomy is the very last option. ➢ Mandibular advancement splints treat snoring and sleep apnea by moving the lower jaw forward slightly, which tightens the soft tissue and muscles of the upper airway to prevent obstruction of the airway during sleep. The tightening created by the device also prevents the tissues of the upper airway from vibrating as air passes over them.
40	C	Continuous positive airway pressure (CPAP). ➢ This is the gold standard treatment for obstructive sleep apnoea (OSA), which may be defined as the cessation of airflow for more than 10 sec in spite of normal respiratory effort. ➢ Patients with OSA often suffer with a host of symptoms including excessive day time sleepiness (daytime somnolence), headaches, poor concentration and hypertension. The CPAP is applied through a face mask or nasal prongs, and the air acts as a pneumatic splint to keep the airway

		open by the positive intraluminal pressure. ➢ CPAP also may be used to treat pre-term infants whose lungs have not fully developed. CPAP treatment involves a CPAP machine, which has three main parts: ➢ A mask or other device that fits over the nose and mouth. ➢ A tube that connects the mask to the machine's motor. ➢ A motor that blows air into the tube. ➢ Some CPAP machines have other features as well, such as heated humidifiers.
41	J	Hitselberger's sign ➢ This refers to paraesthesia of the posterior ear canal, and if present should raise the index of suspicion of an acoustic neuroma. ➢ It is due to compression of the sensory component of the facial nerve in the internal auditory canal by an expanding vestibular schwannoma.
42	L	Schwartze's sign ➢ Reddish-blue discolouration behind the tympanic membrane, typical of otosclerosis, but it is not often seen. It is caused by dilated vessels on the

		promontory of the mucous membrane. ➢ Otosclerosis is a metabolic bone disease exclusive to bone of otic capsule. The increase in metabolism during pregnancy is thought to speed up the process. This produces a slowly progressive conductive hearing impairment. ➢ In some cases, the disease process may also extend from bony tissue to the cochlea itself, causing a mixed conductive and sensorineural hearing loss. ➢ It is inherited in an autosomal dominant fashion with variable penetrance. ➢ Environmental factors implicated in the aetiology of otosclerosis include oestrogens, fluoride and viral infections such as measles.
43	N	Tullio phenomenon ➢ Noise-induced vertigo, dizziness, nausea and/or nystagmus. It was first described in 1929 by the Italian biologist Pietro Tullio after experiments on pigeons. ➢ The aetiology is usually that of a fistula in the middle or inner ear, allowing abnormal sound-

<table>
<tr><td></td><td></td><td>synchronized pressure changes in the semicircular canals.
➢ The opening may be the result of barotrauma (e.g. diving or flying), or may be a side effect of fenestration surgery, syphilis or Lyme disease.
➢ Tullio phenomenon is probably most often seen in patients with superior canal dehiscence syndrome, which is due to the absence of bone over the superior semicircular canal Management involves plugging the superior canal via a middle fossa craniotomy or a transmastoid approach.</td></tr>
<tr><td>44</td><td>H</td><td>Gradenigo's syndrome
➢ Rare complication of acute otitis media, consisting of spreading infection along the petrous apex causing neurological signs which can be remembered using the mnemonic 'EAR.'
• Ear discharge
• Abducens nerve palsy (causes diplopia)
• Retro-orbital pain (due to Trigeminal nerve involvement as the ganglion sits in Meckel's cave adjacent to the petrous apex)</td></tr>
</table>

		➢ Other symptoms can include photophobia, excessive lacrimation, fever, and reduced corneal sensitivity. ➢ Treatment involves high dose antibiotic treatment, both systemic and topical, extended for long periods even if the patient appears to respond adequately to a short regimen. ➢ If the disease is recognised at a later stage, then surgical drainage in the form of apical petrosectomy may be necessary. However, the natural history acute otitis media tends to involve rupture of the tympanic membrane and ear discharge of pus.
45	E	Uncuffed fenestrated. ➢ Fenestrated tubes have small openings on the tube above the cuff (if present). These allow upper airflow and thereby facilitate speech. ➢ Most paediatric tracheostomy tubes are uncuffed. With an uncuffed fenestrated tracheostomy, patients can be ventilated with or without the inner cannula in place. ➢ The tube also aids in the weaning process. General points regarding tracheostomy tubes: Tubes can be plastic (PVC or Silicone) or metal (silver or stainless steel). All have an

		obturator to assist tube insertion. Tubes are available with or without an inner cannula. The inner cannula aids cleaning to prevent tube blockage, but has the disadvantage of reducing the internal diameter (which in turn increases the work of breathing and paradoxically traps secretions.
46	C	Cuffed non-fenestrated. ➢ Cuffed non-fenestrated tubes are used for the first few days after a tracheostomy. The cuff provides an airway seal for effective ventilation and reduces aspiration. ➢ High pressures (above 18 mmHg) can decrease capillary blood flow and cause mucosal ischaemia. ➢ A further disadvantage of a cuffed tube is that it interferes with the swallowing mechanism due to anchorage of the inflated cuff onto the larynx.
47	A	Adjustable flange tubes. ➢ These tubes are suitable for patient with larger necks and increased pretracheal space. Thick neck, bull neck, obese and trauma patients can be assured a secure airway, without the use of endotracheal tubes in tracheal stomas.

		➢ The tight-to-shaft (TTS) cuff facilitates stomal insertion. Adult TTS™ Adjustable Neck Flange Hyperflex Tracheostomy Tubes include a tracheostomy tie and obturator/introducer device. ➢ Adjustable neck flange tracheostomy tubes are intended for temporary use until the proper length fixed neck flange tube can be obtained.
48	L	200 mg - 1% = 10 mg/mL 10% = 100 mg/mL = 200 mg/2 mls
49	A	5 µg - 1% = 10 mg/mL = 10,000 µg/mL = 1:100 10 µg/mL = 1:100,000 5 µg/mL = 1:200,000
50	E	12.5 µg - 1% = 10 mg/mL = 1:100 10 µg /mL= 1:100,000 1:80,000 = 10 µg x 100,000 80,000 = 12.5 µg
51	I	5 mg - 1% lidocaine = 10 mg/ml 5% lidocaine = 50 mg/mL = 50 mg/1000 ul =5 mg/100ul
52	N	Xerostomia. ➢ Common complaint of the elderly leading commonly to speech and eating difficulties as well as halitosis. ➢ Various causes are known including dehydration, diseases affecting the

		salivary glands (e.g. poorly controlled diabetes, Lambert–Eaton syndrome) and often as a result to polypharmacy. ➢ Drugs reduce salivary flow by sympathomimetic or anticholinergic action. Therefore, tricyclics and beta-blockers are amongst the most common implicated agent. Omeprazole is also associated with xerostomia. ➢ Treatment involves finding any correctable causes and removing them if possible. In many cases it is not possible to correct the xerostomia itself, and treatment focuses on relieving the symptoms and preventing cavities. Patients with xerostomia should avoid the use of decongestants and antihistamines, and pay careful attention to oral hygiene. Artificial salivas are often the treatment of choice for xerostomia patients.
53	J	Sialosis (sialadenosis) ➢ Benign condition that causes bilateral painless parotid swelling between the ages of 40–60 years and is equally common in both sexes. ➢ Thought to have an underlying neuropathic aetiology, and is

		therefore seen in diabetics and alcoholics. Any disorder that affects the digestion of food, or its absorption over a prolonged period malnutrition (pellagra or kwashiorkor, cystic fibrosis and pancreatitis, anorexia nervosa and bulimia) can result in sialosis. ➢ One explanation is that the sympathetic nerve supply to the secreting acinar cell is concerned with the production and secretion of zymogen, the precursor of amylase. Because of sympathetic nerve dysfunction, there may be an increase in zymogen storage in the cell, owing to increased production, decreased secretion of the granules or both. ➢ No treatment is required apart from addressing underlying precipitating factors such as poorly controlled diabetes or alcoholism. If the gland is disfiguring, a lateral parotidectomy may be considered but this is quite radical
54	K	Sjögren's. ➢ An autoimmune disorder characterised by xerostomia, bilateral non-tender parotid enlargement and xerophthalmia (keratoconjunctivitis

		sicca). It may be associated with a connective tissue disease such as rheumatoid arthritis or systemic lupus erythematosus. ➢ The xerostomia can be so severe it leads to dysarthria and dysphagia and dysgeusia. ➢ Diagnosis is aided by the presence of SS-A or SS-B autoantibodies, rheumatoid factor or antinuclear antibodies. Diagnosis however is confirmed by the microscopic examination of a minor salivary gland biopsy that demonstrates a focus score of > 1 focus/ 4 mm^2. ➢ Complications of the condition include mastication difficulties, dental decay and oral mucosal discomfort. There is a 10% incidence of lymphoma in patients with Sjögren's syndrome.
55	G	Mucoceles. ➢ Mucocoeles that represent dilatations of minor salivary gland ducts are due to the accumulation of mucous secretions, and mucous extravasations into the connective tissue. ➢ They are the commonest minor salivary gland disorder, and are seen frequently in the lateral aspect of the

		lower lip (60–70%), buccal mucosa, floor of mouth and palate. ➢ Ranulas are mucoceles that occur in the floor of the mouth, and usually involve the major salivary glands. Specifically, the ranula originates in the body of the sublingual gland, in the ducts of Rivini of the sublingual gland, in the Wharton duct of the submandibular gland, and, infrequently from the minor salivary glands at this location. ➢ These lesions are divided into two types: oral ranulas and cervical or plunging ranulas. Oral ranulas are secondary to mucus extravasation that pools superior to the mylohyoid muscle, whereas cervical ranulas are associated with mucus extravasation along the fascial planes of the neck. ➢ With large or recurrent mucoceles surgical excision is the treatment of choice.
56	H	Necrotising sialometaplasia. ➢ Benign, self-healing inflammatory process mainly affecting the minor salivary glands. It presents as a spontaneously appearing painless ulceration/swelling over the hard palate, but may also occur anywhere

		else where salivary gland tissue exists. ➢ There is often surrounding burning sensation, and paraesthesia with systemic features such as pyrexia and malaise. Ulceration never extends to bone and resolution is seen within 90 days, hence the low recurrence rates. ➢ Diagnosis is confirmed by histology that shows acinar necrosis with squamous metaplasia of ductal epithelium. For this reason, it can be misdiagnosed as squamous cell carcinoma leading to unnecessary treatment and associated morbidity.
57	C	Bone conduction hearing aid ➢ This is the best initial device for a professional surfer who suffers with recurrent ear infection and has exostoses. ➢ It is also suitable for patients with a discharging mastoid cavity who requires sound amplification. ➢ Bone conduction hearing aids are generally indicated for meatal discharge, stenosis, or subjective preference for bone conduction reception. ➢ Conventional bone conduction aids had the disadvantage of being bulky and uncomfortable. In addition, some

		sound energy is dissipated through the soft tissue before reaching the skull. Bone anchored hearing aids overcome a few of these drawbacks. ➢ There are two such devices in clinical use: (1) the standard BAHA with a percutaneous titanium screw and (2) the Xomed audient bone transcutaneous conductor, consisting of an encased rare earth magnet implanted completely under the skin and fixed into bone. ➢ The symphonic sound bridge middle ear implant works on the same principle as the Xomed audient. However, the external magnet vibrates a coil that is attached to the incus, hence directly vibrating the ossicles. ➢ In summary a bone conduction aid is suitable in cases where a hearing loss exists in association with an active outer or middle ear disease.
58	H	No device ➢ Many factors influence the choice of hearing aid devices. For instance, the actual degree and nature of the hearing loss dictate the amplification needed. The cause of the hearing impairment will also influence the

type of aid chosen.

- In this question, the patient has only mild hearing loss at one frequency. At least three sub-threshold levels are needed for programming of the digital hearing aids to have any significant benefit in signal to noise ratio.
- The basic components of any hearing aid are a receiver, an amplifier/processor and a sound transmitter. There are two types of signal processing system: analogue and digital.
- In the analogue system, the signal is converted to its electrical analogue at the microphone level, and this is then amplified. The amplified signal is then re-converted to an acoustic sound and passed to an earphone or bone conductor.
- With digital signal processing the analogue sound is converted to its digitally equivalent and then sampled. Each sample is digitally coded, with binary numbers which can then be manipulated mathematically. The number of parameters that can be utilized is greater than those of the analogue system. Therefore the digital hearing ear can be fine-tuned to the

		needs of the patient
59	A	Body worn hearing aid ➢ Body worn (BW) hearing aids are large unattractive aids that are usually worn with a strap around the neck or clipped onto clothing. ➢ However, because of their size they can be made very powerful, and the distance between the microphone and ear piece means that feedback is not a problem, even with high amplification. ➢ Body worn hearing aids are suitable for elderly patients, especially if bed bound or suffering from arthritis. ➢ Syndromic or patients with learning difficulties may also be suitable candidates for this type of hearing amplification device.
60	J	Spectacle hearing aid ➢ This patient has single sided deafness and may have problems determining the direction of sounds because of the head shadow effect. ➢ Spectacle hearing aids involve modifying the spectacle frame to incorporate the aid. The hearing aid may be a standard air conduction aid or a bone conductor for contralateral routing of signal (CROS) in single sided

		deafness. ➢ Here the sound is picked up from the affected side of the head and transferred to the other good side. This helps to reduce the head shadow effect and improves directional perception of sounds. ➢ An alternative to the CROS aid is the BAHA. ➢ Spectacle hearing aids are useful for those who regularly wear glasses, and they can be disguised easily. They are often chosen when there is unilateral profound deafness.
61	H	Spatula misting. ➢ Spatula misting test is useful when no other equipment is available. It involves holding a cold metal spatula (or even a spoon or a mirror) under the nose whilst the mouth remains closed. ➢ The test demonstrates nasal respiration, but gives only a rough approximation of the nasal airflow outwards. Similar information may be obtained by listening to nasal outflow using a stethoscope. ➢ This is particularly useful when assessing children and may help to diagnose nasal obstruction due to a

			mass or even choanal atresia. ➢ Nasal expiratory peak flow has been attempted, but it is uncomfortable since the Eustachian tubes are inflated. It produces excessive mucus in the facemask. ➢ In contrast, nasal inspiratory peak flow involves the use of a peak flowmeter adapted with a nasal mask. It is used in the same way as a peak flowmeter to give information about nasal airway with the patient in their normal environment or whilst taking medications. It is effort dependent and is reduced by conditions such as alar collapse, asthma and COAD.
62	E	Peak flow. ➢ The peak expiratory flow (PEF), also called peak expiratory flow rate (PEFR) is a person's maximum speed of expiration, as measured with a peak flow meter. ➢ It measures the airflow through the bronchi, and thus the degree of obstruction in the airways. ➢ Peak flow testing is the simplest way of assessing pulmonary function and involves blowing into a peak flow meter. Three attempts are made, and the best score is noted. If the result is	

		not within the normal range related to age and height, the test is repeated 15 minutes after administration of salbutamol or terbutaline. A 20% increase in peak flow suggests asthma. ➢ Measurement of PEFR requires training to correctly use a meter and the normal expected value depends on a patient's sex, age and height. Due to the wide range of 'normal' values and high degree of variability, peak flow is not the recommended test to identify asthma. ➢ However, it can be useful in some circumstances. A small proportion of people with asthma may benefit from regular peak flow monitoring. When monitoring is recommended, it is usually done in addition to reviewing asthma symptoms and frequency of reliever medication use. When peak flow is being monitored regularly, the results may be recorded on a peak flow chart. It is important to use the same peak flow meter every time.
63	A	Acoustic rhinometry. ➢ Acoustic rhinometry testing is essential tympanometry of the nose. It employs a sound pulse (150–10,000

		Hz) generated by an electronic click and transmitted in a sound tube to the nose. The sound is reflected by local changes in acoustic impedance, because of changing cross-sectional area with distance. ➢ The reflected sound is picked up by a microphone, and analysed on a computer. The volume at different distances in the nose is then calculated. ➢ Acoustic rhinometry is often confused with rhinomanometry, which is a technique for evaluating nasal patency or obstruction, and airflow by simultaneously measuring transnasal pressure and airway resistance, and pressure-flow characteristics.
64	E	T2 N0 ➢ This type of question requires a very simple exercise in the application of the TNM descriptors upon know facts, the history and sex although useful clinically are less relevant in this exercise, don't get confused! You will have to learn the TNM for larynx, thyroid, nasopharynx sinuses and oral cavity as a minimum. ➢ Staging of melanoma and skin would be useful knowledge. In clinical

		practice reference is always made to ensure accuracy. The salient features are a 3 cm hypopharyngeal cancerous ulcer, the vocal folds were mobile, with no palpable lymph nodes hence T2 N0.
65	G	T3 N0 ➢ The salient features are mass in the left ethmoid sinus invading the orbit but not the extending intracranially and no neck nodes henceT3 N0.
66	K	Treacher–Collins ➢ Abnormality in the first and second pharyngeal arches. ➢ ENT manifestations include microtia, conductive hearing loss, ossicular malformations, pre-auricular sinuses and fistulae, cleft palate, mandibular and midfacial hypoplasia. ➢ Other syndromes associated with a conductive hearing loss include Kartagener's and Goldenhar. In the former, conductive hearing loss is mild and secondary to middle ear effusion. In the latter, the hearing loss is moderate and the patient may require a bone conduction or bone anchored hearing aid. ➢ Turner's syndrome (45XO, due to the absence of a sex chromosome) is

		interesting in that the deafness may be either conductive or sensorineural. Other features of Turners are short stature, infertility, webbing of the neck and a low posterior hairline.
67	D	Branchio-otorenal ➢ Autosomal dominant disorder characterised by abnormalities of the branchial arches, ear and kidneys. It is associated with sensorineural hearing loss and other ENT features such as pre-auricular sinus, dysplastic pinna and branchial fistula discharging mucus on the anterior surface of the neck. Renal abnormalities include agenesis, duplex kidneys and hydronephrosis. ➢ Awareness of branchio-otorenal syndrome means that audiometry is needed for all children presenting with branchial or pre-auricular anomalies. ➢ Other syndromes associated with sensorineural hearing loss include Usher, Pendred, Waardenburg, Alport, CHARGE, Jervell–Lange-Nielsen and Alstrom. ➢ Jervell–Lange-Nielsen syndrome, characterised by prolonged Q–T segment, is particularly important

		because of the history of sudden unexplained syncope or even death in the worse-case scenario. ➢ Management of child with syndromic hearing loss-multidisciplinary team with specialist input from clinical geneticists, audiologists, otolaryngologists, paediatrician and ophthalmologists. ➢ Imaging in the form of high resolution CT scan of the temporal bone and MRI of the inner ear provides invaluable information.
68	C	Beckwith–Wiedemann ➢ Associated with airway abnormalities, and may present with sleep disordered breathing. Airway obstruction is at the level of the tongue base and pharynx mainly because of macroglossia ➢ Other clinical features of this syndrome include ear lobe crease, posterior helical pit, skeletal overgrowth, gastroschisis, hypoglycaemia and renal abnormalities. ➢ The gross macroglossia may be treated surgically with wedge resection to improve cosmesis, but this has no effect on the airway

		obstruction. Children with Beckwith–Wiedemann syndrome may require a nasopharyngeal airway or even a tracheostomy to manage obstructive sleep apnoea. Early mandibular advancement surgery may help to provide some airway relief. ➢ Other conditions associated with airway obstruction at the level of the tongue base/pharynx include Pierre Robin sequence, Sticklers and the craniosynostosis. ➢ Syndromes associated with obstruction at the level of the larynx and trachea include Opitz–Frias (laryngeal cleft) and velocardiofacial (laryngeal webs). ➢ Solitary median maxillary central incisor syndrome (SMMCI) is a rare midline developmental abnormality associated with nasal cavity defects such as piriform aperture stenosis and choanal atresia.
69	C	Horizontal to the left ➢ Horizontal nystagmus is associated with the dysfunction of the lateral semicircular canal. By convention the direction of nystagmus is determined by the direction of the fast phase. A right dead ear means that the slow

		phase would be towards the right. Therefore, the central corrective fast phase would be to the left. In general, a destructive lesion would lead to nystagmus to the opposite side (paralytic nystagmus). ➢ There are two key forms of nystagmus: pathological and physiological, with variations within each type. Nystagmus may be caused by congenital disorders, acquired or central nervous system disorders, toxicity, pharmaceutical drugs or alcohol. ➢ Congenital nystagmus has traditionally been viewed as non-treatable, but medications have been discovered in recent years that show promise in some patients. For example, Baclofen could effectively stop periodic alternating nystagmum, and gabapentin, an anticonvulsant, may cause improvement in some patients. Other drugs found to be effective against nystagmus in some patients include memantine, levetiracetam, 3,4-diaminopyridine, 4-aminopyridine, and acetazolamide. ➢ Several therapeutic approaches, such as contact lenses, drugs, surgery, and

		low vision rehabilitation have also been proposed. ➢ Clinical trials of a surgery to treat nystagmus (known as tenotomy) concluded in 2001. Tenotomy is being performed regularly at the University of Pittsburgh Children's Hospital and by a handful of surgeons around the world. The surgery, developed by Louis F Dell'Osso, aims to reduce the eye shaking (oscillations), which in turn tend to improve visual acuity
70	D	Horizontal to the right ➢ In this scenario, there is no destruction of the labyrinthine. ➢ The nystagmus is due to excessive signalling to the brain from the vestibular system, in other words stimulatory or irritative. This means that there is an imbalance in the inputs going to the brain from the left and right vestibular system. ➢ The slow phase would be to the side that is signalling less, i.e. left. The central corrective fast phase would therefore be to the right. ➢ In general, an irritative or stimulatory lesion would lead to nystagmus to the same side.
71	H	Rotatory geotropic to the right

- Rotatory geotropic nystagmus means that the direction of the nystagmus is towards the earth. It is associated with benign paraxsymal position vertigo. It is always towards the affected ear. Classic BPPV is the most common variety of BPPV. It involves the posterior SCC, and is characterized by the following:
  - Geotropic nystagmus with the problem ear
  - Predominantly rotatory fast phase toward undermost ear
  - Latency (a few secs)
  - Limited duration (< 20 sec)
  - Reversal upon return to upright position
  - Response decline upon repetitive provocation

- Rotational nystagmus also can be described as geotropic and ageotropic. Ageotropic refers to away from the earth. If the head is turned to the right, and the eye rotation is clockwise from the patient's point of view (top half turns to the right and toward the ground), then the nystagmus is geotropic. If the head is turned toward the left, then geotropic

		nystagmus is a counterclockwise rotation. These two terms are useful only when the head is turned.
72	F	Pendular ➢ This type of nystagmus is typical of congenital blindness and lesions in the central tegmental tract. ➢ In contrast to jerk nystagmus (slow and fast phases), it consists of equal oscillations to the right and left like a pendulum. It is sometimes referred to as see-saw nystagmus. ➢ Acquired pendular nystagmus may occur in multiple sclerosis (MS), non-congenital blindness and focal brainstem lesions. ➢ Spasmus nutans is a transient pendular nystagmus that occurs in children; it is associated a head tremor and torticollis. It usually resolves spontaneously in 1–4 years.
73	B	Downbeat ➢ This means that the fast phase is towards the feet. It is part of vertical nystagmus, and is associated with lesion in the lower brainstem. ➢ Upbeat nystagmus (away from the feet) is associated with upper brainstem pathology. ➢ Downbeat nystagmus (DBN) is the

		most common form of acquired involuntary ocular oscillations overriding fixation. It is characterised by slow upward drifts and fast downward phases Slow phase velocity increases on lateral and downward gaze and convergence, although there may be atypical presentations with enhancement of DBN on upward gaze or suppression on convergence. ➢ Craniocervical malformations, cerebellar degeneration, vascular pathology, inflammatory disease and intoxication with lithium or antiepileptic drugs have, among others, been implicated in DBN.
74	K	Tympanosclerosis ➢ Tympanosclerosis (also known as myringosclerosis or intratympanic tympanosclerosis) is a condition caused by calcification of tissues in the middle ear, sometimes resulting in a detrimental effect to hearing. ➢ Myringosclerosis is the term used when just affecting the drum. ➢ Histologically it is calcareous deposits in the fibrous layer of the drum. The pathogenesis involves increased fibroblast activity, resulting in

		deposition of collagen. Calcium phosphate plaques then form in the lamina propria of the tympanic membrane. ➢ Excessive tympanosclerosis may lead to a conductive hearing loss by affecting the compliance of the ear drum. ➢ Treatment involves the use of hearing aid or surgery to remove the sclerotic area. The success rate is variable.
75	E	Enlarged vestibular aqueduct ➢ The vestibular aqueduct is a tiny canal shielded by the temporal bone, one of the densest bones in the body. It houses the endolymphatic duct and sac. ➢ An enlarged vestibular aqueduct (EVA) can be associated with genetic conditions such as Pendred syndrome, which affects thyroid function and hearing, and branchiootorenal syndrome, which affects kidney function and hearing. ➢ It can also be associated with anatomical problems such as Mondini's deformity, when the cochlea develops incompletely. When EVA causes hearing loss or balance symptoms, it is referred to as enlarged

		vestibular aqueduct syndrome (EVAS). ➢ Some people are born with hearing loss, but most hear normally in the first years of life and then notice losses later in childhood, or less commonly in adolescence or early adulthood. Often, this occurs after a minor or major head impact upper respiratory infection or air pressure trauma.
76	E	Epidermoid formation ➢ Epidermoid formation (EF) refers to a small collection of stratified squamous epithelium in the fetal middle ear. In humans, the nest of cells appears between the 10th and 33rd gestational week and then disappears by an unknown mechanism. ➢ The postpartum persistence of these cells has been suggested to be the source of congenital cholesteatoma. Support for this theory is based on the observation that the epidermoid formations are found around the middle ear cavity but predominantly in the anterosuperior epitympanum at the junction of the Eustachian tube with the middle ear, in exactly the same position where the majority of congenital cholesteatomas originate.

		➢ Although the EF is highly plausible explanation for the origin of congenital cholesteatoma, the direct demonstration has not yet been done.
77	I	Retraction pocket theory ➢ This theory is generally accepted as the most common pathogenic mechanism in primary acquired cholesteatoma. According to this theory, the pars flaccida, or occasionally the pars tensa, retracts into the middle ear because of negative middle ear pressure, inflammation or both. ➢ Early retraction pockets may be asymptomatic or associated with mild conductive hearing loss whilst chronic pockets are associated with the retention of keratin as a result of disordered epithelial migration. ➢ The continuous accumulation of keratin, presumably as a result of dysfunctional epithelial migration in the retraction pocket, leads to the development of acquired cholesteatoma. ➢ Recent preliminary temporal bone studies suggest that in retraction pockets which appear to result from chronic otitis media, fetal type

		epithelial hyperplasia may contribute to the development of cholesteatoma by the direct invasion of hyperplastic bands of squamous epithelium into the middle ear.
78	C	Basal hyperplasia theory ➢ This theory states that epithelial cells from the keratinising epithelium of the pars flaccida could invade the subepithelial space and form an attic cholesteatoma. ➢ Subsequent experimental studies have confirmed that the basement membrane dissolves focally: pseudopodia from the basal cell layer seem to break the basal lamina allowing keratinocyte invasion. The entrapped cells keratinise and form inclusion cysts that may expand and form cholesteatoma. ➢ Recent preliminary temporal bone studies are compatible with these observations. This fetal type epidermis was present in varying lengths on the tympanic membrane and deep ear canal and displayed hyperplastic bands (rete ridges) extending into subepidermal tissue which sometimes penetrated the collagen layer of the tympanic

		membrane to enter the middle ear. ➢ Severe chronic otitis media, with inflammatory exudates, glandular metaplasia or tympanosclerosis, was present in the middle ears with fetal type epithelium. This fetal type of epidermal hyperplasia was also seen in retraction pockets.
79	H	Migration theory ➢ Squamous epithelium migrates from the margin of a tympanic perforation into the middle ear cleft causing a secondary acquired cholesteatoma. There is also experimental evidence for this theory in the animal model. ➢ However, if this theory is correct, one might expect a much higher incidence of acquired cholesteatoma considering the incidence of tympanic membrane perforation associated with infection. ➢ The epithelial migration theory is also relevant to congenital cholesteatoma. It states that the fetal tympanic annulus plays a major role in control of proliferation of skin in the external ear canal. If the annulus fails to produce a stop signal in early embryological development, ectodermal tissue grows from the ear

		canal into the middle ear and produces a congenital cholesteatoma. ➢ Furthermore, *in vitro* studies suggest that epidermoid cells from the cerebellopontine angle exhibit migratory properties similar to those of cholesteatoma cells from the middle ear and mastoid cavity. The migration theory may explain the occurrence of congenital cholesteatoma in the posterior and inferior parts of the middle ear, close to the site of the embryonic tympanic ring but it does not explain why the anterosuperior region is the most common site of congenital cholesteatoma. The putative 'stop signal' has not yet been identified.
80	J	Squamous metaplasia theory ➢ It has been suggested that the non-keratinising middle ear mucosa could undergo a metaplastic transformation into keratinising epithelium under the pressure of dried pus. ➢ The metaplastic epithelium grows because of the accumulation of keratin, and recurrent infection leads to perforation of the tympanic membrane resulting in the typical appearance of attic cholesteatoma.

			➢ This theory is supported by the observation that the pluripotent middle ear epithelium could be stimulated by inflammation into a metaplastic stratified squamous epithelium with keratinisation. ➢ Furthermore, biopsies from the middle ear mucosa of children with otitis media with effusion occasionally display islands of keratinising epithelium. ➢ Extreme vitamin A deprivation could cause metaplasia, but is rare in humans. Furthermore, there is no direct histological or experimental evidence that these mechanisms lead to cholesteatoma formation.
81	B	4	(M2+V1+E1) ➢ The Glasgow coma scale (GCS) is a reliable and universally comparable way of recording the conscious state of a person. Three types of response are measured and added together to give an overall score. The lower the score the lower the patient's conscious state. A score of below 8 suggests the patient requires airway support. The lowest possible GCS (the sum) is 3 (deep coma or death), while the highest is 15 (fully awake person).

		The Glasgow Coma scale:
		• Best Motor Response (M) -6 grades (Apply varied painful stimulus: ear lobe pinch, sternal rub, nail-bed pressure)
		  • No response to pain.
		  • Extensor posturing to pain-decerebrate posture.
		  • Abnormal flexor response to pain-decorticate posture.
		  • Withdraws from pain.
		  • Localising response to pain.
		  • Obeying command.
		• Best Verbal Response (V) -5 grades (Record best level of speech).
		  • No verbal response.
		  • Incomprehensible speech: Moaning but no words.
		  • Inappropriate speech: Random or exclamatory articulated speech.
		  • Confused conversation: Patient responds to questions in a conversational manner but some disorientation and confusion.
		  • Orientated
		• Best eye response (E) -4 grades
		  • No eye opening.
		  • Opening to response to pain

		to limbs as above. • Eye opening in response any speech. • Spontaneous eye opening.
82	L	14 (M6+V4+E4)
83	J	12 (M5 +V3+E4)
84	H	Rhinophyma ➢ Severe form of long-standing acne rosacea, and results from hypertrophy of the sebaceous glands at the tip of the nose; it is not a neoplasm. ➢ It presents as a pink, lobulated mass over the nose with superficial vascular dilation; it mostly affects men past middle age. ➢ The condition is also much more common in men than in women and in caucasians compared to black men. ➢ The cause of rhinophyma is unknown, though it is thought to be associated with the organism Demodex follicularis. ➢ Interestingly, patients seek advice mainly because of nasal or visual obstruction, rather than the unsightly appearance of the enlargement. ➢ Treatment consists of paring down the bulk of the tissue with a sharp knife or carbon dioxide laser, allowing the area to re-epithelialise.

		Sometimes, the tissue is completely excised and the raw area skin-grafted.
85	D	Nasal dermoid ➢ The most common congenital nasal masses. Unlike other craniofacial dermoids, the nasal lesions can present as a cyst, a sinus or a fistula and may have an intracranial extension. ➢ Many nasal dermoids present at birth but some are not found until later in childhood or even adulthood when they become symptomatic. ➢ They constitute nearly 3% of all dermoids and contain both ectodermal and mesodermal elements such as hair follicles and sebaceous glands. ➢ Usually, nasal dermoids terminate in a single subcutaneous tract, which can sometimes have hair at the opening. They may secrete sebaceous material or pus and become intermittently inflamed. Connection with the central nervous system has been variably reported to occur from 4-45% and therefore should be investigated with both CT and MR. ➢ Associated congenital anomalies occur in 5-41% of cases which include aural

		atresia, mental retardation, spinal column abnormalities, hydrocephalus, hypertelorism, hemifacial microsomia, albinism, corpus callosum agenesis, cerebral atrophy, lumbar lipoma, dermal cyst of the frontal lobe, coronary artery anomaly, cleft lip and palate, tracheoesophageal fistula, cardiac, genital, and cerebral anomalies. There is no known syndromic association of these anomalies. ➢ A widely accepted theory of dermoid sinus cyst development is the prenasal space theory. During normal development a projection of dura protrudes through the fonticulus frontalis or inferiorly into the pre-nasal space. If this projection persists, the dura can remain attached to the epidermis, and result in trapped ectodermal elements. ➢ Dermoid cysts are managed surgically either excised directly on the dorsal surface of the nose or via an open rhinoplasty procedure.
86	A	Basal cell carcinoma (BCC) ➢ BCC is an epithelial malignant tumour with a low malignant potential, consisting of cells arise from the basal

epidermis layer.

- The diagnostic histological features, common for all types of the tumour, are basaloid cells with a thin pale cytoplasm, surrounding round or oval nuclei with a rough granulated chromatin pattern
- Basal cell carcinoma has been divided into four types: nodular, pigmented, superficial and morpheaform.
  - *Nodular Basal Cell Carcinoma*

Nodular BCC (the most common form) is characterized by the appearance of a flesh-toned nodule that, is covered with inflamed small blood vessels and is round in shape.

- *Pigmented Lesion Basal Cell Carcinoma*

Pigmented lesion BCC is much darker in coloration than the nodule type. It is the blue-brown-black hue that identifies this type of BCC.

- *Superficial Basal Cell Carcinoma*

The third and least common type of BCC is the superficial type. It is red in coloration with a scaly texture. It can easily be confused with other skin anomalies such as eczema or psoriasis.

		• *Morpheaform (Sclerosing)* This type of BCC looks like a scar with an indurated yellow to white plaque with an indistinct border. Ulceration and crusting are usually absent but his variety has an aggressive growth pattern, and invasion of muscle, nerve, and bone may be seen. Morpheaform BCC is particularly insidious because of its benign scar-like appearance. Differential diagnosis of morpheaform BCC includes scarring and localized superficial scleroderma (morphea). MOHs surgery is recommended to ensure clear margins.
87	F	MRI Stir sequence ➢ Parotid gland tumours should be assessed with an ultrasound scan and cytology in the first instance. However, prior to operation a more detailed investigation is required especially if deep lobe invasion is suspected. ➢ The best MRI sequence for this is the Short Tau inversion Recovery, which suppresses fat and helps identify the facial nerve. In general, MRI is a medical imaging technique used to visualise detailed soft tissue structures

		by using of the property of nuclear magnetic resonance to image nuclei of atoms inside the body. ➢ MRI provides good contrast between the different soft tissues of the body, which makes it especially useful in imaging the brain, muscles, the heart, and cancers compared with other medical imaging techniques such as computed tomography (CT) or X-rays. ➢ In contrast to CT scans or traditional X-rays, MRI does not use ionising radiation.
88	D	Gadolinium-enhanced MRI scan ➢ Vestibular Schwannoma is suspected with asymmetrical sensorineural hearing loss. Imaging modality of choice is contrast-enhanced MRI on T1 weighted images. ➢ Although this is the gold standard it is time and labour intensive. Many centres are now using T2 images, which supply better anatomical detail but have a higher false negative rate. Some centres now check urea and electrolytes before administering Gadolinium.
89	E	MRI non-echo planar diffusion weighted ➢ The traditional management of patients who had a combined

		approach tympanoplasty for cholesteatoma is to go back and re-examine the mastoid 9–12 months later for reccurrence or residual disease. ➢ The advent of diffusion weighted MRI has now allowed definition of 2 mm cholesteatomas. ➢ In some centres (especially in Belgium) a non EPI diffusion weighted scan is performed instead of a second look procedure. ➢ In summary, the use of MRI imaging may promote the use of canal wall up procedure and obviate the need for routine second look procedures.
90	C	FDG PET-CT ➢ Metastatic head and neck cancer with unknown primary is a possible presentation of a neck mass. A thorough ENT examination and CT of neck and chest should be performed, or MRI neck and CT chest. If these investigations do not help point to a primary site, then a FDG PET CT should be performed. ➢ This is a nuclear scan that looks for high mitotic activity. The likely sources of the unknown primary are the tonsils, tongue base and post nasal

		space. A blind biopsy can be performed of these sites. However, if the results come as normal than the PET scan will have to be delayed as the operative site lights up on the scan giving a false positive. Therefore, if the PET scan is readily available in the department than it should be performed first, but if it is not than one should consider blind biopsies. ➢ PET-CT scanning is also useful for disease surveillance following definitive treatment. ➢ In summary, FDG-PET is helpful for the detection of occult primary tumours and distant metastases but it is not reliable enough for the detection of occult lymph node metastases.
91	H	MRI T2 image ➢ A T2 weighted MRI scan is the best option as CSF produced a high signal (water is white on T2 water images, and dark on T1). ➢ High resolution fine cut CT scans of the skull base can be useful in defining bony dehiscence and site of CSF leak. However, a bony defect is not the same as the site of CSF leak. ➢ Intra-thecal contrast is not used in the UK. Intra-thecal fluorecin 30 minutes

		before repair procedure may be helpful. ➢ T_2-weighted scans are another basic type. Like the T_1-weighted scan, fat is differentiated from water, but in this case fat shows darker, and water lighter. For example, in the case of cerebral and spinal study, the CSF (cerebrospinal fluid) will be lighter in T_2-weighted images. These scans are therefore particularly well suited to imaging oedema.
92	H	Tramadol ➢ Tramadol is used to treat moderate to severe pain. It is a centrally acting synthetic analgesic of the aminocyclohexanol group with opioid-like effects. ➢ It appears to act by modifying transmission of pain impulses via inhibition of noradrenaline and serotonin re-uptake and also by weakly binding to μ-opioid receptors. ➢ Side effects include many of the gastrointestinal side effects of opioid agonists. ➢ Tramadol has other therapeutic uses, including treatment for Rheumatoid arthritis, restless legs syndrome and fibromyalgia. While its action is not

		typical of other opioids, the drug is a synthetic analog of the phenanthrene alkaloid codeine. ➢ The euphoria and respiratory depression of opioids are mainly caused by the μ_1 and μ_2 receptors; the addictive nature of tramadol, as well as other opioids, is due to these effects, but tramadol's serotonergic and noradrenergic effects may contribute to possible dependence as well.
93	G	Paracetamol ➢ The apparent selectivity of paracetamol may be due to inhibition of COX-2 dependent pathways that are proceeding at low rates. This is consistent with the similar pharmacological effects of paracetamol and the selective COX-2 inhibitors. ➢ Side effects include rash, thrombocytopenia, leucopenia, liver and renal damage. When taken in overdose the liver conjugation becomes inundated, causing paracetamol to be metabolised by an alternative pathway. This results in a toxic metabolite, N-acetyl-p-benzoquinone imine (NABQI), which is

		itself usually inactivated by glutathione, preventing any harm. Any process which depletes glutathione (e.g. alcohol excess) worsens this effect.
94	A	Aspirin ➢ Reye's syndrome is a very rare condition that causes serious liver and brain damage. If it is not treated promptly it may result in permanent brain injury or death. ➢ Almost all recorded cases of Reye's syndrome have happened in children, but adult cases have also occurred. ➢ The exact cause of Reye's syndrome is unknown, but there is evidence that two factors may contribute towards children developing the condition. Previous viral infection – most children who developed Reye's syndrome were recovering from a viral infection, usually either influenza or chickenpox. Many children who developed Reye's syndrome had previously taken aspirin to treat the symptoms of their viral illness.
95	C	Thy 3 ➢ *Thy 3 (indeterminate)* This can fall into either I) follicular

lesion/suspected follicular neoplasm. II) cytological findings not allowing clear categorisation. These cases should be discussed in the MDT meeting if a therapeutic procedure is being considered. While some of these will be tumours, many will be shown to be hyperplastic nodules on surgical excision.

- Fine needle aspiration cytology is the diagnostic investigation of choice in the many thyroid units. It is also quick to perform and obtain results. Sensitivity of 95% and specificity of 86% have been reported.
- The cytological classification of thyroid aspirates consists of five categories (THY 1 to THY 5). However, there are a few points worth noting. Whilst the diagnosis of papillary carcinoma is simple, the distinction between benign and malignant follicular neoplastic cells is impossible because the diagnosis of follicular carcinoma is dependent on seeing vascular or capsular invasion on a histological section.
- When the cytology is reported as follicular, a diagnostic thyroid lobectomy is often required. Fine

		needle aspiration may result in a sampling error, especially with very small <1 cm, very large >4 cm, haemorrhagic nodules or nodules in a multinodular goitre. Such problems can be reduced by multiple sampling and ultrasound guided aspiration cytology.
96	B	Thy 2 ➢ *Thy 2 (benign)* Non-neoplastic, e.g. colloid nodule or thyroiditis. However, subsequently up to 10% can be proven to be malignant therefore a repeat sample should be taken in 3–6 months. If a Thy2 is obtained again it is reasonable to observe the lesion. In high clinical risk group cases, the decision to proceed to lobectomy may be made even with a benign FNAC diagnosis. For completion, the following should be noted: ➢ *Thy 1 (inadequate sample)* Non-diagnostic. Therefore, should be repeated. It is more common if the lesion is <1cm in size. ➢ *Thy 4 (suspicious)* These lesions are suspicious but not diagnostic of malignancy: papillary, medullary, anaplastic carcinoma or

		lymphoma. Where Thy 4 assessment has been given because of the absence of material for immunocytochemistry (medullary carcinoma) or flow cytometry (lymphoma), the aspirate should be repeated. *Thy 5 (malignant)* Diagnostic of malignancy, demonstrating unequivocal features of papillary, medullary or anaplastic carcinoma, lymphoma or metastatic tumour.
97	N	Wilcoxon matched-pairs test ➢ In this question there is one group of subject (1 sample) reporting two sets of data that are non-parametric. Here we have a sample measured under two conditions and the null hypothesis is that there is no tendency for the outcome on one condition to be higher or lower that the other. The alternative hypothesis is that the outcome on one condition tends to be higher or lower that the other. ➢ Wilcoxon matched-pairs test is an equivalent of the paired *t*-test, which is more powerful and is used if the differences are normally distributed.

		The Wilcoxon test is almost as powerful as a *t*-test and in practice the difference is not great. ➢ The sign test is similar in power to the Wilcoxon for very small samples, but as the sample size increases, the latter becomes much more powerful since the Wilcoxon test uses more of the information.
98	H	One sample (paired) Student's *t*-test ➢ One group of subject (1 sample) whose weights (parametric variables) are being tested before and after a special diet, comparing average blood pressures between a group of men and women. ➢ The choice of statistical test is fundamental to data interpretation. When selecting the relevant-test one must consider the type of data collected as well as the aim of analysis. ➢ All statistical tests are either parametric (i.e. they assume that the data were sampled from a particular form of distribution, such as a normal distribution) or non-parametric (i.e. they do not assume that the data were sampled from a particular type of distribution). Non-parametric tests

<table>
<tr><td></td><td></td><td>look at the rank order of the values (which one is smallest, which one comes next and so on).
➢ In general, parametric tests are more powerful than non-parametric ones and so should be used if at all possible. Parametric testing (e.g. student t-test) is performed on data that is normally distributed, independent of each other and has a constant variance and is described by mean and sd.
➢ Non-parametric testing (e.g. Wilcoxon match pairs) is for data not normally distributed (e.g. pain, examination scores), described by median and range usually needs a large n to get significance. In summary the one-sample (paired) t-test compares two sets of observations on a single sample (tests the hypothesis that the mean difference between two measurements is zero).</td></tr>
<tr><td>99</td><td>L</td><td>Two sample (unpaired) Student's t-test
➢ Here you have two groups or samples (male & female) but only one variable (BP) which is normally distributed. Essentially similar to the above but compares two independent t samples drawn from the same population. The</td></tr>
</table>

		unpaired t method tests the null hypothesis that the population means related to two independent, random samples from an approximately normal distribution are equal. ➢ Power is calculated as the power achieved with the given sample sizes and variances for detecting the observed difference between means with a two-sided type I error probability of (100–CI%)%. ➢ The unpaired t-test should not be used if there is a significant difference between the variances of the two samples. Note that the unpaired *t*-test is often more robust to use the non-parametric. Mann–Whitney test as an alternative method in the presence of unequal variances.
100	K	Spearman's rank correlation coefficient ➢ The number of consultations and the skills score are both integer variable taking a reasonable range of values. They cannot be assumed to follow a continuous normal distribution. Spearman correlation coefficient is correct because it is a valid way to determine an association between two non-normal measures. ➢ Paired *t*-test is inappropriate because

			the data are not normally distributed and a comparison of two paired groups is not required. ➢ McNemar is inappropriate because the data are not binary (two-category) and a comparison of two paired groups is not required. ➢ There are several other numerical measures that quantify the extent of statistical dependence between pairs of observations: these are discussed at correlation and dependence. The most common of these is the Pearson product moment correlation coefficient.

CHAPTER 2

Paper 2

EMI Questions (Q1-Q100)

For each stem, select one correct answer option.

Theme: Facial nerve palsy

Options for Questions 1–5:

A Active squamous chronic otitis media
B Bell's palsy
C Facial nerve neuroma
D Facial nerve transaction
E Guillain–Barré syndrome
F Herpes zoster
G Lyme disease
H Melkersson–Rosenthal syndrome
I Moebius syndrome
J Myasthenia gravis
K Primary Sjögren's
L Sarcoidosis
M Squamous cell carcinoma
N Transverse temporal bone fracture

For each of the following cases, select the single most likely diagnosis. Each option may be used once, more than once or not at all.

1. A 25-year-old male motorcyclist presents with a left facial nerve palsy following an accident that involved him landing on the back of his head. He also has bleeding from his left ear, and right beating nystagmus associated with ipsilateral profound hearing loss.
2. A 45-year-old man presents with right sided facial nerve palsy (House–Brackmann grade 4). He states that prior to the facial weakness, he had a dull ache in the right ear. He also had a history of itching and discharge from both ears. Examination revealed normal tympanic membranes and canals with flaky skin on both sides.
3. A 55-year-old woman presents generalised weakness and bilateral facial nerve palsies. After ruling out raised intracranial pressure, the medical registrar proceeded to a lumbar puncture. The result shows raised CSF protein.
4. A 65-year-old male alcoholic presents with a 5-day history of right facial nerve palsy, and bruising on the face and body. Examination of his ear revealed purulent discharge obscuring the view of the tympanic membrane.
5. A 55-year-old woman presents with tiredness, that gets worse towards the end of the day. Examination reveals bilateral facial nerve weaknesses associated with bilateral ptosis.

Theme: Hoarse voice

Options for questions 6–10

A	Candidiasis of the larynx
B	Carcinoma of the bronchus
C	Carcinoma of the oesophagus
D	Chronic laryngitis
E	Hypothyroidism
F	Keratosis of the vocal folds
G	Laryngeal papillomatosis
H	Laryngocele
I	Squamous cell carcinoma of larynx
J	Vocal cord granuloma
K	Vocal cord nodules
L	Vocal cord palsy

For each of the following cases, select the single most likely diagnosis. Each option may be used once, more than once or not at all.

6. A 52-year-old man presents with a 1-month history of a hoarse voice. He takes oral antacid therapy for indigestion, and denies any dysphagia.

7. A 22-year-old woman presents with a 2-month history of a hoarse voice. She is an amateur singer.

8. A 55-year-old man presented with an intermittent neck swelling associated with hoarseness, cough and discomfort. Examination of the neck did not reveal any palpable masses, but indirect laryngoscopy revealed fullness in the upper left hemilarynx.

9. A 55-year-old man presents with almost no voice. He was operated on three times for whitish lesions on his vocal folds. Biopsies taken at each operation revealed no evidence of malignancy.

10. A 65-year-old man presents with a 4-week history of hoarseness. He smokes twenty cigarettes a day, and has been short of breath and wheezing for some time. His GP recently prescribed him a steroid inhaler. On examination, his throat is red with white patches. Flexible nasendoscopy revealed a whitish lesion on the right vocal cord. Both cords move normally. There was no cervical lymphadenopathy.

Theme: Conditions of the mouth

Options for Questions 11–14

A Behçet's disease
B Crohn's disease
C Erythema Multiforme
D Geographical tongue
E Hereditary angio-oedema
F Koplik's spots
G Median Rhomboid glossitis
H Mucous membrane pemphigoid
I Osler-Weber-Rendu syndrome
J Pemphigoid
K Pemphigus vulgaris
L Peutz–Jeghers syndrome

For each of the following cases, select the single most likely diagnosis. Each option may be used once, more than once or not at all.

11. A 48-year-old woman presents with oral ulcers. Immunological investigations reveal antibodies to desmoglein 3.

12. A 50-year-old man presents with oral ulcers after taking sulphonamides.

13. A 48-year-old woman presents with oral blisters and ulcers. Immunological investigations reveal antibodies to a basement membrane protein.

14. A 21-year-old male presents with a swollen tongue and lips, which settled with C1 esterase concentrate.

Theme: Hearing loss

Options for Questions 15–19

- A Auditory neuropathy
- B Ménière's disease
- C Noise induced hearing loss
- D Otitis media with effusion
- E Otosclerosis
- F Pendred syndrome
- G Presbyacusis
- H Waardenburg syndrome type 1
- I Waardenburg syndrome type 1I
- J Waardenburg syndrome type 1II
- K Waardenburg syndrome type 1V

For each of the following cases, select the single most likely diagnosis. Each option may be used once, more than once or not at all.

15. A 35-year-old female presents with a gradual painless reduction in hearing on the left side during her pregnancy. There were no other otological symptoms, or significant past medical history. On examination, her ears were normal. Weber's lateralized to the left, and Rinne's test was negative. Pure tone audiogram shows a 40 dB conductive hearing loss.

16 A 23-year-old female presents with difficulty listening to speech, but has no problems with music. She feels her symptomology is worse in the left. Pure tone audiogram is just within normal thresholds. Otoacoustic emissions are present, but stapedial reflexes are absent in her left ear.

17. A 4-year-old boy presents with normal hearing at birth, that has had a stepwise bilateral sensorineural deterioration in his hearing. He is found to be hypothyroid and has goitre.

18 A 45-year-old female presents with a low frequency sensorineural hearing loss noted on pure tone audiogram. She has normal tympanometry and stapedial reflexes.

19. A 67-year-old male presents with bilateral high frequency sensorineural hearing loss.

Theme: Surgical indications

Options for Questions 20–24:

A Adenoidectomy
B Adenotonsillectomy
C Antral washout
D Balloon sinuplasty
E Excision lymph node biopsy
F Functional endoscopic sinus surgery
G Incision lymph node biopsy
H MDT Discussion
I Myringotomy and insertion of grommets
J No surgery indicated
K SMD Inferior turbinates
L Tonsillectomy
M Turbinate surgery

For each of the following cases, select the single most appropriate treatment. Each option may be used once, more than once or not at all.

20 A 4-year-old boy from Bangladesh presents with a two-month history of rapidly increasing left anterior triangle mass. Ultrasound reveals multiple, enlarged, conglomerating roundish lymph nodes that are hypoechoic. Chest X-ray, Heaf test, and full blood count are equivocal. The paediatricians have asked for a biopsy to rule out tuberculosis.

21. An 8-year-old boy presents with recurrent tonsillitis. His mother gives a history of heavy snoring, but no witnessed apnoeic episodes. There is no daytime

somnolence or irritability. He has had four attacks of tonsillitis a year for the last 2 years.

22. A 26-year-old male presents with recurrent acute left maxillary sinusitis. CT scan shows opacification within left antrum.

23. A 4-year-old female presents with nasal blockage, snoring and witnessed episodes of obstructive sleep apnoea. She is irritable in the morning and has poor concentration throughout the day.

24. A 46-year-old man presents with a 3-month history of a rapidly enlarging level 2 lymph node. Has had night sweats, fever and weight loss. The node is painful when he drinks alcohol. ENT examination is otherwise normal. Fine needle cytology of the lymph node shows atypical lymphocytes but cannot rule out lymphoma.

Theme: Neck dissections

Options for Questions 25–28:

A Bilateral selective neck dissection
B Modified radical neck dissection type 1
C Modified radical neck dissection type II
D Modified radical neck dissection type III
E Radical neck dissection
F Selective neck dissection level I– III
G Selective neck dissection level II–IV
H Selective neck dissection level I–IV
I Selective neck dissection level II–V

J Selective neck dissection II,III,IV, VI

For each of the following cases, select the single most appropriate neck dissection. Each option may be used once, more than once or not at all.

25. A 55-year-old man presents with a four-month history of a painful ulcer on the lateral border of his tongue. Examination and biopsy confirms a 3cm squamous cell carcinoma. Enhanced CT scan did not reveal any involved cervical lymph nodes.

26. A 67-year-old man presents with difficulty swallowing. Examination reveals a large ulcerative lesion in the left piriform fossa, and palpable level II and III lymph nodes. He was unable to shrug his shoulder on the left side. MR of the neck reveals metastatic invasion of the sternocleidomastoid and internal jugular.

27. A 47-year-old man presents with a 4cm thyroid swelling. Examination reveals a 4cm solitary lesion, and a 2 cm level III lymph node. FNAC confirms the presence of papillary carcinoma.

28. A 60-year-old woman presents with hoarseness. Examination and biopsy reveals a 4cm supraglottic squamous cell carcinoma. A CT scan reveals that the lesion crosses the midline, but no cervical lymphadenopathy was detected.

Theme: Common ENT surgical instruments

Options for Questions 29–30:

A Anterior commissure laryngoscope
B Boyle's–Davis
C Cattle's speculum
D Freer's elevator
E Gwynne Evans dissector
F Jolls retractor
G Mollison's pillar retractor
H Negus laryngoscope
I St Claire currette
J Thudicum speculum
K Tilley Henkel forceps
L Travers retractor
M Trousseau tracheal dilators
N Tumarkin aural speculum

For each of the following surgical tasks, select the single most appropriate tool. Each option may be used once, more than once or not at all.

29. Used to dissect the tonsil from its muscular attachments.

30 Used to help reinsert a displaced tracheostomy tube.

Theme: Management of laryngeal carcinoma

Options for Questions 31–34:

A Chemoradiotherapy
B Chemotherapy

C Cricothyroidotomy
D Partial laryngectomy
E Pharyngolaryngectomy
F Proton beam therapy
G Radiotherapy
H Surveillance
I Total laryngectomy
J Tracheostomy
K Transoral laser

For each of the following cases, select the single most appropriate management. Each option may be used once, more than once or not at all.

31. A 47-year-old man presents with a hoarse voice. Microlaryngoscopy reveals a lesion on the left vocal fold, extending to the anterior commissure. Biopsy shows squamous cell carcinoma.

32. A 47-year-old female smoker presents with a hoarse voice. Flexible nasendoscopy reveal a whitish lesion on the right vocal fold. A vocal fold biopsy reveals grade II dysplasia.

33. A 56-year-old male smoker presents with hoarseness. Flexible nasoendoscopic examination reveals a keratotic lesion on the right vocal fold, extending into the anterior commissure and crossing the midline. The right vocal cord was immobile. A biopsy revealed squamous cell carcinoma. CT imaging revealed the lesion extending into the both table of the thyroid lamina.

34. A 65-year-old man presents with difficulty in breathing. He is unable to finish a sentence. Recently he was diagnosed with T3 squamous cell carcinoma of larynx, and is currently receiving chemoradiotherapy.

Theme: Rhinitis

Options for Questions 35–39:

A Allergic Rhinitis
B Atrophic rhinitis
C CSF rhinorrhoea
D Drug induced rhinitis
E Food induced rhinitis
F Hormonal rhinitis
G Idiopathic rhinitis
H Non allergic eosinophilic rhinitis
I Non allergic occupational rhinitis

For each of the following cases, select the single most likely diagnosis. Each option may be used once, more than once or not at all.

34. A 27-year-old pregnant smoker presents complaining of nasal blockage and rhinorrhoea.

35. A 40-year-old male air traffic controller complains of severe nasal blockage and rhinorrhoea when out working in the cold. His symptoms persist to a lesser degree when not working.

36. A 25-year-old asthmatic woman presents with severe rhinorrhoea after taking aspirin

37. A 50-year-old woman presents with nasal crusting and blockage. She is known to have Wegener's granulomatosis.

38. A 17-year-old female presents with hay fever and asthma complains of nasal and conjunctival pruritus, sneezing and rhinorrhoea.

Theme: Sinus anatomy

Options for Questions 40–42:

A Agger Nasi cell
B Anterior osteomeatal Unit
C Concha Bullosa
D Ethmoid Infundibulum
E Haller cell
F Hiatus Semilunaris
G Lamina Papyracea
H Maxillary sinus ostium
I Onodi cell
J Uncinate

For each of the following statements, select the single most likely corresponding anatomical structure. Each option may be used once, more than once or not at all.

40. 3-Dimensional cleft between uncinate medially and lamina papyracea laterally.

41 Functional area bounded by middle turbinate medially and uncinate bone laterally.

42. Is formed by the 1st lamella of the lateral nasal wall.

Theme: TNM staging

Options for Questions 43–44:

A T1N0M0

B T1N1M0

C T1N1aM0

D T1N1bM0

E T2N0M0

F T2N1M0

G T3N0M0

H T3N1M0

I T4N0M0

J T4N1M0

For each of the following cases, select the single most appropriate TNM stage. Each option may be used once, more than once or not at all.

43. A 45-year-old man presents with a 6-month history of a neck lump. Examination reveals a nodule in the right thyroid lobe, and a 2 cm, level 5 lymph node. Ultrasound scan revealed a 2cm lesion in the thyroid gland, and FNAC suggests papillary carcinoma.

44. A 45-year-old man presents with a 6-month history of a neck lump. Examination reveals a nodule in the right thyroid lobe, and a 2 cm, level 4 lymph node. Ultrasound scan revealed a 1cm lesion in the thyroid gland, and FNAC suggests papillary carcinoma.

Theme: NICE guidelines on the management of otitis media with effusion

Options for Questions 45–49:

A Adenoidectomy
B Adenotonsillectomy
C Antibiotics
D Insert Grommets
E Insert grommets and perform adenoidectomy
F Otovent balloon
G Prescribe topical decongestants
H Prescribe topical steroids
I Recommend hearing aids
J Repeat hearing test in 3 months
K Repeat hearing test with 6 week time interval
L Tonsillectomy

For each of the following cases, select the single most appropriate management. Each option may be used once, more than once or not at all.

45 A 12-year-old Down's child presents with otitis media with effusion, proven over multiple time points, resulting in reduced hearing.

46. A 4-year-old boy presents with first presentation of bilateral conductive hearing loss secondary to glue ear.

47. A 4-year-old boy presents for the second time with a unilateral 20 dB conductive hearing loss secondary to otitis media with effusion. His other ear has normal hearing.

48. A 5-year-old girl presents with 40 dB conductive hearing loss bilaterally, found after 3 months of watchful waiting. She frequently suffers from upper respiratory tract infections and nasal blockage.

49. A 5-year-old boy presents with cleft palate and glue ear, proven over multiple time points and resulting in 40 dB conductive hearing loss.

Theme: Drug constituents

Options for Questions 50–52:

A Azelastine
B Betamethasone, neomycin
C Betamethasone, sodium phosphate
D Dexamethasone, neomycin, acetic acid
E Fluticasone furoate
F Fluticasone propionate
G Gentamycin, hydrocortisone
H Gramicidin, framycetin sulphate dexamethasone
I Iodoform paraffin bismuth
J Iodoform, benzoin, storax
K Ipratropium bromide
L Lidocaine, adrenaline (epinephrine)
M Lidocaine, phenylephrine
N Mometasone furoate

For each of the following pharmaceutical agents, select the chemical constituent(s) present. Each option may be used once, more than once or not at all.

50. Avamys.

51. Rinatec.

52. Whitehead's varnish.

Theme: Parapharyngeal space neoplasms

Options for Questions 53–54:

A Metastatic lesion
B Salivary gland lesion
C Neurogenic lesion
D Lymphoma

For each of the following cases, select the single most likely diagnosis. Each option may be used once, more than once or not at all.

53. A 49-year-old man presents complaining of asymmetrical tonsils. On examination he was found to have a medially displaced right tonsil. A CT scan report stated that he had a solid lesion in the pre-styloid compartment of his parapharyngeal space.

54. A 49-year-old man presents complaining of asymmetrical tonsils. On examination he was found to have a medially displaced right tonsil. A CT scan report stated that he had a solid lesion in the post-styloid compartment of his parapharyngeal space.

Theme: Salivary gland tumours

Options for Questions 55–59:

A Acinic cell carcinoma
B Adenocarcinoma

C Adenoid cystic carcinoma
D Adenolymphoma (Warthin's tumour)
E Carcinoma ex-pleomorphic adenoma
F Haemangioma
G Lymphangioma
H Lymphoma
I Monomeric adenoma
J Mucoepidermoid carcinoma
K Neurofibroma
L Pleomorphic adenoma
M Ranula
N Salivary mucocele

For each of the following histological descriptions, select the single most likely corresponding lesion. Each option may be used once, more than once or not at all.

55. Benign lesion containing foci of mucus, hyaline and cartilage.

56. A cystic lesion without a true epithelial lining.

57. A cystic lesion lined by a double layer of epithelium.

58. Is described histologically as having a Swiss cheese pattern.

59. Is divided histologically into 3 grades: Low, intermediate and high.

Theme: Sleep disorders in adults

Options for Questions 60–64:

A Central sleep apnoea

B Cheyne–Stokes respiration
C Idiopathic hypersomnolence
D Insomnia
E Narcolepsy
F Night terrors
G Normal variant
H Obstructive sleep apnoea
I Periodic limb movement disorder
J Upper airways resistance syndrome

For each of following cases, select the single most likely diagnosis. Each option may be used once, more than once or not at all.

60. A 35-year-old male presents with excessive day time somnolence. Polysomnography shows no apnoeic episodes, and 2 hypopnoeic episodes per hour. However, there are frequent snoring related arousals. Oesophageal manometry during sleep shows progressive increase in oesophageal pressure terminating in arousal.

61. A 45-year-old male presents complaining of difficulty initiating sleep, excessive daytime somnolence, and frequent nocturnal awakenings. Polysomnography shows no apnoeas/hypopnoeas. However, there are 5 movements of the flexors of his lower limb every hour.

62. A 16-year-old male presents with a 6-month history of severe day time somnolence. He has frequent day time naps but they do not make him feel more refreshed. He sleeps 12 hours at night and wakes up,

when forced, still feeling tired. Polysomnography is normal.

63. A 65-year-old female presents with heart failure, who complains of daytime somnolence and poor night's sleep. Polysomnography shows apnoea with no thoracic or abdominal movement.

64. A 32-year-old female presents with daytime somnolence and poor night's sleep. She describes vivid dreams whilst falling asleep or on awakening. She can fall asleep very easily and without control during the day. Polysomnography shows REM sleep within 5 minutes of sleep.

Theme: Complications of acute sinusitis

Options for Questions 65–69:

- A Adhesions within the nose
- B Cavernous sinus thrombosis
- C Cerebral abscess
- D Extradural abscess
- E Orbital abscess
- F Orbital cellulitis
- G Pott's Puffy tumour
- H Preseptal cellulitis
- I Subperiosteal abscess
- J Sinus thrombosis

For each of the following cases, select the single most likely diagnosis. Each option may be used once, more than once or not at all.

65. A 6-year-old girl presents with history of upper respiratory tract infection. Examination revealed warm red oedematous eyelid, conjunctival injection with chemosis and restricted ocular motility with diplopia. Her condition did not improve following intravenous broad spectrum antibiotic therapy

66. A 3-year-old boy presents with history of upper respiratory tract infection, and has developed red swollen eye lid. There is no proptosis or chemosis and vision is normal.

67. A 6-year-old boy presents with a painful doughy swelling on his forehead following acute sinusitis.

68. A 6-year-old boy presents with bilateral proptosis, severe headache and loss of sensation over forehead and eyes bilaterally.

69. A 7-year-old girl presents with acute sinusitis and periorbital cellulitis and drowsiness. Examination reveals splinter haemorrhages and neck stiffness.

Theme: Topical aural preparations

Options for Questions 70–74:

A Betnesol
B Betnesol–N
C Betnovate
D Canesten
E Ciprofloxacin
F Gentisone
G Gentisone HC

H Locorten-Vioform
I Ofloxacin
J Otomize
K Otosporin
L Sofradex
M Synalar ointment

For each of the following chemical constituents, select the single mostly likely corresponding topical aural preparation. Each option may be used once, more than once or not at all.

70. Dexamethasone, framycetin and gramicidin.

71. Hydrocortisone, neomycin and polymxin B.

72. Dexamethasone, neomycin and acetic acid.

73. Flumetasone and clioquinol.

74. Clotrimazole.

Theme: Difficulty swallowing

Options for Questions 75–78:

A Achalasia of the oesophagus
B Gastro-oesophageal reflux
C Globus pharyngeus
D Goitre
E Myaesthenia gravis
F Oesophageal cancer
G Oesophageal candidiasis
H Oesophageal foreign body
I Pharyngeal pouch

J Recurrent laryngeal nerve palsy
K Stroke
L Unilateral hypoglossal nerve palsy

M Vagus nerve palsy

For each of the following cases, select the single most likely diagnosis. Each option may be used once, more than once or not at all.

75. An 80-year-old man presents with sudden onset in difficulty in swallowing. He lives in a nursing home, and was recently diagnosed with dementia. The nurse accompanying him stated that he did not have any previous swallowing problems and had eaten breakfast a few hours ago.

76. A 44-year-old housewife presents to her GP complaining of a feeling of a lump in her throat for the past 6 months. She pointed at the level of her thyroid cartilage, but had no pain in her throat. Clinical examination was normal although she was slightly overweight.

77. A 23-year-old male drug addict presents to Accident and Emergency with a history of pain and difficulty in swallowing over the past week. He had a chronic cough, and weight loss, and had been treated previously in the department for abscesses at the injection sites.

78. A 35-year-old woman presents with increasing difficulty in swallowing over the previous 3 months. This become worse as a meal progressed, and has

been associated with 14 lb (6.5 kg) of weight loss. She also complains of general tiredness and weakness.

Theme: Dizziness and vertigo

Options for Questions 79–82:

A Acoustic neuroma
B Acute vestibular failure
C Benign paroxysmal positional vertigo (BPPV)
D Meniere's disease
E Migraine
F Multiple sclerosis
G Psychogenic
H Stroke
I Vertebrobasilar ischaemia

For each of the following cases, select the single most likely diagnosis. Each option may be used once, more than once or not at all.

79. A 60-year-old woman presents to her GP with a history of intermittent spinning sensation lasting between 6-12 hours at a time. This was usually preceded by a feeling of fullness in the ear, together with unilateral hearing loss and tinnitus.

80. A 70-year-old man presents with an intermittent spinning sensation which began 2 months ago after a minor head injury. He described attacks lasting for 1–2 minutes usually when turning over to the right side in bed.

81. A 40-year-old woman presents with a feeling of 'wooziness' whenever she went to a shopping mall. She had to sit down to recover and often complained of tingling in her fingers.

82 A 50-year-old man presents with acute onset of a debilitating spinning sensation associated with nausea and vomiting. This occurred shortly after an upper respiratory tract infection, and slowly improved over several days.

Theme: Facial pain/headache

Options for Questions 83–84:

A Acute sinusitis
B Atypical facial pain
C Chronic sinusitis
D Classic migraine
E Cluster headache
F Common migraine
G Demylinating condition, such as multiple sclerosis
H Motor neuron disease
I Otitis media
J Sphenopalatine ganglion neuralgia
K Temporal arteritis
L Temporomandibular joint dysfunction
M Tension headache
N Trigeminal neuralgia

For each of the following cases, select the single most likely diagnosis. Each option may be used once, more than once or not at all.

83. A 45-year-old woman presents with intermittent severe temporofacial pain. Each episode begins with severe pain in and around the right ear, radiating across the right side of the face and down to the right jaw. More recently she describes severe pain when touching her lower lip on the right and can now not bear to put on lipstick. Her clinical and neurological examination is normal apart from observing an internuclear ophthalmoplegia.

84. A 25-year-old woman presents complaining of marked episodic frontal headache associated with phonophobia and nasal congestion, but no rhinorrhoea or droopy eyes. Each episode lasts for hours and takes her to bed. A 2-week course of antibiotic and nasal decongestants were ineffective.

Theme: Micro-organisms relevant to otolaryngology

Options for Questions 85–89:

A Actinomyces
B Atypical Mycobacterium
C Bacteroides spp
D Borrelia burgdorferi
E Fusobacterium necrophorum
F Klebsiella rhinoscleromatis
G Pseudomonas aeruginosa
H Rhinosporidium seeberi
I Rochalimaea (Bartonella) henselae
J Staphylococci

K Streptococcus milleri

For each of the following cases, select the single most likely infective organism. Each option may be used once, more than once or not at all.

85. A 6-year-old girl presents with suppurative and necrotising granulomatous lymphadenitis with stellate abscesses. She owns a cat.

86. A 25-year-old woman presents with severe left frontal headache of 2-days duration. She vomited twice in the last hour, and now appears drowsy. She is normally fit and well but recently been on a scuba diving holiday. On examination she has neck stiffness and mucopus in both nostrils.

87. A 45-year-old male Mexican presents with mucopurulent rhinorrhoea. Examination reveals inflamed nasal mucosa and intranasal nodules.

88. A 14-year-old boy presents with fever, arthralgia and facial nerve palsy following an adventure holiday in Sweden.

89. A 45-year-old Thai man from presents with rhinorrhoea, and foul smelling discharge from his nose. He wife says that his nose has been growing. He also has some nodules on his hands.

Theme: Cranial nerves

Options for Questions 90–94:

A Olfactory nerve

B Optic nerve
C Occulomotor nerve
D Trochlear nerve
E Trigeminal nerve
F Abducens nerve
G Facial nerve
H Audiovestibular nerve
I Glossopharyngeal nerve
J Vagus nerve
K Spinal Accessory
L Hypoglossal nerve

For each of the following anatomical statements, select the single most appropriate cranial nerve. Each option may be used once, more than once or not at all.

90. The shortest of the cranial nerves and is capable of regeneration.

91. The only cranial nerve that exits from the dorsal aspect of the brainstem.

92. Innervates stylopharyngeus.

93. Sends secretomotor fibres to the parotid gland.

94. Innervates the anterior belly of digastrics.

Theme: Diagnostics

Options for Questions 95–97:

A Left labyrinthitis obliterans
B Left Ménière's disease
C Left otosclerosis

D Left superior semicircular canal dehiscence
E Left Unilateral peripheral vestibular deficit
F Left vestibular schwannoma
G Normal (no abnormality)
H Right labyrinthitis obliterans
I Right Ménière's disease
J Right otosclerosis
K Right superior semicircular canal dehiscence
L Right unilateral peripheral vestibular deficit
M Right vestibular schwannoma

For each of the following investigation results, select the single most likely diagnosis. Each option may be used once, more than once or not at all.

95. Electrocochleography done bilaterally shows summating potential to action potential ratio of 0.5 on left and 0.2 on right.

96. CT scan shows ossification of the labyrinthine membrane on the left, and MRI does not show the membrane.

97. Pure tone audiogram shows left conductive hearing loss. Tympanometry is normal and ear examination reveals no abnormality.

Theme: Statistical testings

Options for Questions 98–100:

A Chi-squared ($\chi 2$) test
B Fisher's exact-test
C Friedman test

D F-test
E Kruskal–Wallis test
F Mann–Whitney U test
G McNemar
H One Sample (paired) Student's t-test
I One-way analysis of variance (ANOVA)
J Pearsons correlation coefficient
K Spearman's rank correlation coefficient
L Two sample (unpaired) Student's t-test
M Two-way analysis of variance (ANOVA)
N Wilcoxon matched pairs test

For each of the following data sets, select the single most suitable statistical test. Each option may be used once, more than once or not at all.

98. To assess whether likelihood to pass the state surgery exam is greater in Boston training programme applicants compared to applicants from elsewhere.

99. Correlation of the blood pressure and age between a group of men and women.

100. To determine whether air conduction thresholds changes with increasing age.

Answer Keys to Chapter 2 EMIs

1	N	Transverse temporal bone fracture ➢ Road traffic accident resulting in facial nerve palsy, profound hearing loss and nystagmus strongly suggests a temporal bone fracture. Severe frontal or occipital force tends to lead to transverse fracture whilst a lateral force over the mastoid or temporal squama results in a longitudinal fracture. ➢ Cochlear and vestibular structures are usually damaged in a transverse fracture, producing a profound sensorineural hearing loss and severe ablative vertigo. The presence of right nystagmus means that the vestibular system is dysfunctional in that there is a reduced activity from the left side (or excessive stimulation from the right). ➢ A transverse fracture of the temporal bone is not as common as a longitudinal fracture (20% vs 80%, respectively). ➢ Signs and symptoms of a longitudinal fracture include bleeding into the ear canal and tympanic membrane laceration, haemotympanum, external auditory canal fractures, ossicular

		chain disruption that produces a conductive hearing loss. ➢ If facial nerve palsy occurs immediately after a longitudinal temporal bone fracture, it is most likely due to a segment of bone pressing on the nerve. Exploratory tympanotomy with facial nerve decompression may reverse the nerve palsy. Both transverse and longitudinal fractures of the temporal bone may also occur simultaneously.
2	B	Bell's Palsy ➢ The information give in this case is quite non-specific and does not fit with a definitive cause for the facial nerve palsy. ➢ Any of the condition listed can cause facial nerve palsy. Bell's palsy would be a provisional diagnosis until the patient is fully investigated and no cause found. Therefore, Bell's palsy is a diagnosis of exclusion and may be defined as idiopathetic (cryptogenic) unilateral facial nerve palsy. ➢ The condition is usually self-limiting but tends to respond to steroids therapy. ➢ Bell's palsy is the most common acute mononeuropathy with a rapid onset of

		partial or complete palsy that often occurs overnight. ➢ It is thought that an inflammatory condition, probably precipitated by a virus, leads to swelling of the facial nerve within its bony canal. Corticosteroids have been found to improve outcomes while anti-viral drugs have not. ➢ Most cases recover spontaneously and achieve near-normal to normal functions. Many show signs of improvement as early as 10 days after the onset, even without treatment. The eye must be protected from drying and debris otherwise the cornea will become permanently damaged resulting in impaired vision.
3	E	Guillain–Barré syndrome ➢ Acute inflammatory demyelinating polyneuropathy affecting the peripheral nervous system because of an auto-immune response directed against Schwann cell membranes. ➢ Classically, there is paralysis, starting in the extremities and moving towards the central trunk. The lower cranial nerves are affected more frequently than the upper. In addition to motor weakness, sensory disturbances and

		reduced proprioception may occur. ➢ Of the six different subtypes of Guillain–Barré syndrome, acute inflammatory demyelinating polyneuropathy (AIDP) is the most common form. ➢ The Miller Fisher variant is paralysis occurring in the reverse (antegrade) direction and accounts for approximately 5% of cases. It usually affects the eye muscles first and presents with the triad of ophthalmoplegia, ataxia, and areflexia. Acute panautonomic neuropathy is the rarest variant of GBS, sometimes accompanied by encephalopathy. ➢ The most common symptoms at onset are related to orthostatic intolerance, as well as gastrointestinal and sudomotor dysfunction. Parasympathetic impairment (abdominal pain, vomiting, constipation, ileus, urinary retention, dilated unreactive pupils, and loss of accommodation) may also be observed.
4	A	Active squamous chronic otitis media ➢ This patient may have had a head injury followed by an infection in the ear; the bruising could be as a result of

		deranged clotting from chronic liver disease. However, when there is purulent discharge from the ear, one always has to rule out the presence of cholesteatoma. ➢ A significant amount of discharge from the ear usually means that the middle ear is involved because of the mucosal lining and therefore there must be a perforation in the tympanic membrane. In the past, a chronic discharge of pus in the presence of a perforated tympanic membrane was referred to as chronic suppurative otitis media (CSOM). However, pus is not always present and chronic otitis media (COM) may be better classified as active mucosal COM (old CSOM), inactive mucosal COM (perforation), active squamous COM (cholesteatoma) and inactive squamous (retraction). ➢ Another entity is healed COM where there is a permanent abnormality of the *pars tensa*, but the ear has no tendency to become active because the tympanic membrane is intact and there is no retraction pocket.
5	J	Myasthenia Gravis ➢ Autoimmune neuromuscular disease which causes fluctuating muscle

		weakness characterized by premature fatigability. ➢ It is caused by autoimmune antibodies which most commonly block the nicotinic acetylcholine receptors at the neuromuscular junctions, inhibiting the excitatory effects of the neurotransmitter acetylcholine on nicotinic receptors throughout neuromuscular junctions. ➢ Myasthenia gravis must be distinguished from congenital myasthenic syndromes that can present similar symptoms but offer no response to immunosuppressive treatments. ➢ Symptoms include ptosis, diplopia, dysphagia and dysarthria. ➢ Treatment is with cholinesterase inhibitors, immunosuppressants or in rare cases thymectomy. It can be occasionally life threatening due to myasthenic crisis which affects the respiratory muscles
6	D	Chronic laryngitis ➢ Laryngitis causes hoarse voice or complete loss of voice because of irritation to the vocal folds. Dysphonia is the medical term for a vocal disorder, of which laryngitis is one

		cause. ➢ Laryngitis is categorized as acute if it lasts less than a few days. Otherwise it is categorized as chronic, and may last over 3 weeks. The chronic form of disease occurs mostly in middle age and is much more common in men than women. ➢ The aetiology is multifactorial encompassing vocal abuse, smoking and gastro-oesophageal reflux. In its milder form the vocal folds are inflamed. In more extreme forms there is marked oedema and swelling known as Reinke's oedema. ➢ Symptoms include hoarseness or dysphonia, dry sore burning throat, coughing, (which can be a symptom of, or a factor in causing laryngitis), lump sensation and stridor. ➢ Initial therapy aims to reduce risk factors, for example smoking cessation, coupled with voice therapy and anti-reflux medications. In severe cases of Reinke's oedema, surgery can be utilised to remove the oedematous matrix of the vocal cord.
7	K	Vocal cord nodules ➢ These arise from vocal misuse and are otherwise known as 'singers' or

		'screamers' nodules. Typically, they will appear on the junction of the anterior and middle third of the vocal cords, where contact is most forceful. ➢ The nodules appear as symmetrical swellings on both sides of the vocal cords. Nodules reduce or obstruct the ability of the vocal folds to create the rapid changes in air pressure which generate human speech. ➢ Symptoms include hoarseness, painful speech production, frequent vocal breaks, and reduced vocal range. Vocal fold nodules develop mostly in adult females and children of both sexes. Nodules are the most common cause of a hoarse voice in children. ➢ Persons who are often susceptible are those who use their voice constantly in a loud environment, for example, teachers, cheerleaders, politicians, actors, preachers, singers, and military instructors. ➢ Treatment is conservative with speech and language therapy. Large firm nodules may need surgical excisions along with speech therapy.
8	H	Laryngocele ➢ Laryngoceles arise from the laryngeal saccule and is usually seen in glass

		blower or wind instrument players. ➢ It refers to a congenital anomalous air sac communicating with the cavity of the larynx, which may bulge outward in the neck causing Bryce's sign (a hissing or gurgling sound produced by manual pressure on an external laryngocele). ➢ It may also be acquired due to continual forced expiration producing increased pressures in the larynx which leads to dilatation of the laryngeal ventricle. It is also seen in people with chronic obstructive airway disease. ➢ Laryngoceles may expand internally to fill the vestibule or may pass externally through the thyrohyoid membrane. They are occasionally associated with ventricular carcinoma. ➢ Lateral neck X-ray may show an air-filled sac but CT imaging is more helpful. ➢ The main complication is airway obstruction, especially if the laryngocele becomes infected. ➢ The safest treatment is excision with the upper half of the thyroid cartilage on the affected side.
9	F	Keratosis of the vocal folds ➢ Keratosis or hyperkeratosis of the larynx is a localized hyperplasia of the

		epithelium. Grossly, it appears as a white or grayish-white elevated area that may be smooth but usually is irregular and wrinkled. ➢ Microscopically, keratosis is recognized by an increase in the size of the squamous epithelial layer, especially of the cornified portion. Both Keratosis and leukoplakia of the vocal folds are premalignant lesions. ➢ The aetiology remains unknown, but factors which contribute to their onset and development are thought to include smoking and voice misuse and abuse. ➢ The cessation of smoking when the individual is a smoker, and/or the elimination of voice misuse and abuse when such prevails may result in a reduction or elimination of the lesions Patients with hyperplasia, keratosis, leukoplakia, hyperplasia, dysplasia and carcinoma *in situ* should be carefully followed up, as invasive carcinoma may develop many years after the initial diagnosis.
10	I	Squamous cell carcinoma of the larynx ➢ This patient has laryngeal carcinoma until proven otherwise. The main risk factor associated with squamous cell

		carcinoma of the larynx is smoking. ➢ Candidiasis would be part of the differential diagnosis, although he could have both conditions simultaneously. ➢ Squamous cell carcinoma accounts for 95% of all malignancy tumours of the larynx and tend to occur at the junction of the anterior 1/3 and 2/3 of the vocal cord (the same site of vocal cord nodules). For this reason, anyone with hoarseness for more than 3 weeks needs a laryngoscopic examination. ➢ In this way laryngeal cancer can be detected and treated early, thereby preventing significant morbidity and mortality. ➢ Candidiasis is common in patients on steroid inhalers or who are immunocompromised such as HIV and diabetic patients.
11	K	Pemphigus ➢ Pemphigus is an autoimmune condition whereby IgG attacks desmoglein -3. Desmoglein is the glue that allows epithelial cells to bind to one another. Therefore, in this disease the epithelial cells separate from one another causing blisters. ➢ Patients present with blisters that

		often burst and turn into ulcers before. In pemphigus, autoantibodies form against desmoglein. When autoantibodies attack desmogleins, the cells become separated from each other and the epidermis becomes 'unglued', a phenomenon called acantholysis. This causes blisters that slough off and turn into sores. In some cases, these blisters can cover a significant area of the skin.
12	C	Erythema multiforme ➢ Erythema multiforme is a condition caused by IgM deposition in the superficial microvasculature of the skin and mucous membranes. It results in target shaped rash on the skin that starts peripherally and resolves in 10 days. ➢ It is a skin condition of unknown cause, possibly mediated by deposition of immune complex (mostly IgM) in the superficial microvasculature of the skin and oral mucous membrane that usually follows an infection or drug exposure. ➢ It is a common disorder, with peak incidence in the second and third decades of life. The condition varies from a mild, self-limited rash (E.

		multiforme minor) to a severe, life-threatening form known as erythema multiforme major that also involves mucous membranes. This severe form may be related to Stevens–Johnson syndrome. ➢ The mild form is far more common than the severe form. ➢ Diagnosis is confirmed by biopsy. ➢ The mild form usually presents with mildly itchy, pink-red blotches, symmetrically arranged and starting on the extremities. It often takes on the classical 'target lesion' appearance, with a pink-red ring around a pale centre. Resolution within 7–10 days is normal.
13	J	Pemphigoid ➢ Pemphigoid is a group of uncommon and rare autoimmune blistering skin diseases. Pemphigoid is similar to pemphigus, but, unlike pemphigus, pemphigoid does not feature acantholysis. ➢ Pemphigoid is more common than pemphigus, and is slightly more common in women than in men. Pemphigoid is a disease where IgG targets BP-1. This is a protein that connects epithelium to the dermis and

		is present in the basement membrane. Therefore, the epithelium peels away from the underlying dermis. The blisters are tougher and last longer than in pemphigus.
14	E	Hereditary angio-oedema ➢ Hereditary angio-oedema is an autosomal dominant disorder involving antibody formation against C1 esterase inhibitor. Angio-oedema may be congenital or acquired. ➢ Hereditary angioedema (types I and II) is characterized by local swelling in subcutaneous tissues and is caused by a deficiency of the C1 esterase inhibitor, a protein of the complement system, a part of the immune system. Some mutations produce low levels of C1 inhibitor (type I); others produce normal levels of ineffective C1 protein (type II). ➢ C1 inhibitor is needed to control the coagulation cascade in blood clotting, the complement cascade in the immune system, and the contact cascade which is also part of the inflammatory system. Deficiency of C1 inhibitor causes hereditary angioedema types I and II. ➢ Hereditary angioedema type III has

		separate pathogenesis, being caused by mutations in F12 gene coding for a serine protease called Factor XII. It mimics allergic angio-oedema with minor trauma as the trigger. In the majority of hereditary cases C1esterase inhibitor levels are reduced. ➢ Oedema of the lips and throat can last from hours to days. The potent vasodilator bradykinin plays a role in angio-oedema and therefore the condition may be a side effect of ACE inhibitors such as enalapril. Consumption of NSAIDS or vasodilator foods such as alcohol or cinnamon can increase the probability of an angio-oedema episode in susceptible patients.
15	E	Otosclerosis ➢ This patient has a conductive hearing loss with a normal appearing tympanic membrane. Otosclerosis can result in conductive and/or sensorineural hearing loss. ➢ Most of the implicated genes are transmitted in an autosomal dominant fashion with variable penetrance. ➢ The primary form of hearing loss in otosclerosis is conductive hearing loss which usually begins in one ear but

		eventually affect both ears with a variable course. ➢ On audiometry, the hearing loss is characteristically low-frequency, with higher frequencies being affected later. ➢ Sensorineural hearing loss (SNHL) has also been noted in patients with otosclerosis; this is usually a high-frequency loss, and usually manifests late in the disease. The causal link between otosclerosis and SNHL remains controversial. ➢ Post mortem studies show that as many as 10% of people may have otosclerotic lesions of their temporal bone, but apparently never had symptoms warranting a diagnosis. ➢ Caucasians are the most affected race, with the prevalence in the Black and Asian populations being much lower. In clinical practice otosclerosis is encountered about twice as frequently in females as in males, but this does not reflect the true sex ratio. Usually noticeable hearing loss begins at middle-age, but can start much sooner. ➢ The most likely diagnosis from the selection above is otosclerosis. This is a clinical diagnosis based on progressive hearing loss, often with a family

		history. ➢ Presbyacusis Willisii is associated with this condition and relates to improved hearing of speech in noisy environments. ➢ Classical otosclerosis presents with a conductive hearing loss, normal tympanic membrane and absent stapedial reflexes. The pure tone audiogram can often show a reduction in bone conduction at 2 k Hz, known as Carhart's notch. Surgical treatment involves replacing the stapes with a piston.
16	A	Auditory Neuropathy ➢ Auditory neuropathy (AN) is a variety of hearing loss in which the outer hair cells within the cochlea are present and functional, but sound information is not faithfully transmitted to the auditory nerve and brain properly. A neuropathy usually refers to a disease of the peripheral nerve or nerves, but the auditory nerve itself is not always affected in Auditory Neuropathy Spectrum Disorders. ➢ Auditory neuropathy is diagnosed when a person has present Otoacoustic Emissions and/or Cochlear Microphonics in combination with

		absent or abnormal Auditory Brainstem Response. Patients with Auditory Neuropathy Spectrum Disorders have to date never been shown to have normal middle ear muscle reflexes at 95 dB or less despite having normal otoacoustic emissions. ➢ This condition is little understood. It may be due ineffective inner hair cells, the connection of inner hair cells to the auditory nerve or the nerve itself. Since the outer hair cells are not affected otoacoustic emissions are not effected. Stapedial reflexes are dependent on functioning inner hair cells transmitting sound to the auditory nerve and therefore are absent. ➢ Patients often complain of difficulty hearing speech that is out of proportion to the pure tone audiogram. It can present at birth or in teenage years and there is often a family history.
17	F	Pendred syndrome ➢ Pendred syndrome is an autosomal recessive condition that presents with either bilateral sensorineural hearing loss at birth, or the hearing loss that develops in a step-wise fashion during childhood.

		➢ It is a genetic disorder leading to congenital bilateral sensorineural hearing loss and goitre with occasional hypothyroidism. ➢ There is no specific treatment, other than supportive measures for the hearing loss and thyroid hormone supplementation in case of hypothyroidism. ➢ The hearing loss of Pendred's syndrome is often present from birth, and language acquisition may be a significant problem if deafness is severe in childhood. The hearing loss typically worsens over the years, and progression can be step-wise and related to minor head trauma. ➢ In some cases, language development worsens after head injury, demonstrating that the inner ear is sensitive to trauma in Pendred syndrome; this is as a consequence of the widened vestibular aqueducts. ➢ Vestibular function varies in Pendred syndrome and vertigo can be a feature of minor head trauma. ➢ Goitre is present in 75% of all cases.
18	B	Ménière's disease ➢ The symptoms of Ménière's are variable; not all sufferers experience

		the same symptoms. These include; Attacks of rotational vertigo that can be severe, incapacitating, unpredictable, and last anywhere from minutes to hours, but generally no longer than 24 hours. ➢ For some sufferers however, prolonged attacks can occur, lasting from several days to several weeks, often causing the sufferer to be severely incapacitated. ➢ This combines with an increase in volume of tinnitus and temporary, albeit significant, hearing loss. Hearing may improve after an attack, but often becomes progressively worse. ➢ Nausea, vomiting, and sweating sometimes accompany vertigo, but are symptoms of vertigo, and not of Ménière's; Fluctuating, progressive, unilateral (in one ear) or bilateral (in both ears) hearing loss, usually in lower frequencies. ➢ For some, sounds can appear tinny or distorted, and patients can experience unusual sensitivity to noises; Unilateral or bilateral tinnitus; A sensation of fullness or pressure in one or both ears. This relates to endolymphatic hydrops which has been implicated in

		the pathophysiology of Ménière disease. ➢ The typical attacks of vertigo may be explained in terms of the longitudinal drainage theory which involves endolymph draining too rapidly from the cochlear duct. The endolymph overfills the endolymphatic sinus and overflows into the utricle, stretching the cristae of the semicircular canals causing the attacks.
19	G	Presbyacusis ➢ Presbyacusis is age related hearing loss related to damage of cochlear hair cells. It affects men more than women. ➢ Hearing loss begins at the age of 18 and is progressive. It is made worse by environmental exposure however, is distinct from noise induced hearing loss, which often presents with unilateral disease and a drop at 4 k Hz. ➢ It is defined as a progressive bilateral symmetrical age-related sensorineural hearing loss. The hearing loss is most marked at higher frequencies. Hearing loss that accumulates with age but is caused by factors other than normal aging is not presbycusis, although differentiating the individual effects of multiple causes of hearing loss can be

		difficult. ➢ Over time, the detection of high-pitched sounds becomes more difficult, and speech perception is affected, particularly of sibilants and fricatives. The microscopic changes seen in this condition are hair cell degeneration of the cochlea and giant stereo ciliary degeneration.
20	E	Excision lymph node biopsy ➢ With this history and ultrasonographic findings tuberculosis would be high on the differential diagnosis. Therefore, a chest X-ray and Heaf test should be carried out. If these did not point to a diagnosis of TB, the entity could be atypical tuberculosis. ➢ This could be nearly fully cured if completely excised without the need for further medical treatment. Therefore an excision biopsy would be diagnostic and at the same time curative. Incision biopsy involves removing part of the node and this may be adequate in many situations e.g. for suspicious skin lesions or suspected lymphoma. ➢ A needle biopsy involves inserting a needle into a node to obtain the sample and is the preferred initial

		sampling method for most head and neck lumps in adults but not children.
21	J	No surgery indicated ➢ This child does not meet the SIGN criteria for tonsillitis for recurrent tonsillitis. Although the child snores there is no evidence of sleep apnoea, which would be an indication for adenotonsillectomy. Therefore there is no indication for surgery. ➢ SIGN recommends surgery for recurrent acute tonsillitis that is disabling to life with more than seven attacks in a year, or five attacks a year for last 2 years, or three attacks a year for the last 3 years. ➢ Surgery would be indicated if there is clear evidence of obstructive sleep apnoea, suspicion of cancer or two episodes of peritonsillar abscesses. ➢ Tonsillectomy is occasionally done for access to other structures such as a long styloid process causing Eagle's syndrome or for excision of a 2nd branchial pouch sinus involving the tonsillar fossa.
22	F	FESS ➢ This gentleman has recurrent acute sinusitis. There may be a nidus of infection that remains unresolved or an

		anatomical defect that predisposes his left maxillary sinus to recurrent infections. It is important to clear out any source of infection from this sinus and restore anatomical, physiological drainage. Therefore, a FESS would be more appropriate. ➢ Functional endoscopic sinus surgery (FESS) has now become the mainstay in the surgical treatment of sinusitis and nasal polyps, including bacterial, fungal, recurrent acute and chronic sinus. The complications associated with FESS are significantly reduced because of surgical experience and the use of navigation system which is used to better correlate surgical anatomy with pre-operative CT imaging. CT-navigation assistance in sinus surgery is used to improve anatomical identification and avoid damage to vital structures such as the brain and eyes.
23	B	Adenotonsillectomy ➢ This child is suffering from sleep disordered breathing which represents a spectrum of conditions involving simple snoring, high upper airway resistance, obstructive hypoventilation and obstructive sleep apnoea.

		➢ Primary snoring is involves turbulent airflow and vibration of pharyngeal structures. Noisy breathing as a result of snoring is therefore sterter which is distinctly different from stridor, which is due to laryngotracheal obstruction. ➢ Upper airway resistance syndrome (UARS) is characterised by increased respiratory effort, frequent arousal, no gas exchange abnormalities and a prolonged pulse transit time. ➢ In obstructive hypoventilation syndrome, there is continuous partial obstruction, oxygen desaturation and hypercarbia. ➢ Obstructive sleep apnoea syndrome is characterised by snoring, cessation of airflow, continued respiratory effort and oxygen desaturation. ➢ Predisposing factors in children for sleep disordered breathing include craniofacial abnormalities, space-occupying lesions and neuromuscular disorders. ➢ Diagnosing sleep disordered breathing is made on history, examination and investigation. ➢ Investigations include one or more of the following: polysomnography, pulse oximetry, oesophageal manometry,

		radiology and fibreoscopy. ➢ Treatment of sleep disordered breathing depends on the underlying cause and the options are: ➢ Adenotonsillectomy ➢ Nasopharyngeal airway ➢ Nasal continuous positive airway pressure ➢ Tracheostomy ➢ Osteotomies to correct facial deformities. ➢ Failure to manage sleep disordered breathing adequately may result in cardiopulmonary complications such as pulmonary hypertension, cor pulmonale, dysrhythmias, cardiorespiratory failure and intracranial hypertension.
24	G	Incision lymph node biopsy ➢ This gentleman just needs a diagnosis. It is likely he has lymphoma, but the type and grade are also unknown. This data can sometimes be gained by cytology. However, when the results do not confirm this a biopsy is necessary. ➢ Treatment would be chemotherapy so nothing will be gained by complete surgical excision, whilst the risks of

		surgery will greatly increase. Therefore, incisional biopsy will suffice, although in most case the surgeon may take out a whole node.
25	F	Selective neck dissection level I– III ➢ Level III is defined clinically as the lymph nodes between the hyoid and the cricoid. Surgically it the lymph nodes between the carotid bifurcation and the point where the omohyoid crosses the internal jugular vein. ➢ The cricoid cartilage is the only complete ring of cartilage around the trachea. The function of the cricoid cartilage is to provide attachments for the various muscles, cartilages, and ligaments involved in opening and closing the airway and in speech production. Because of it texture, location and size, the cricoid is a very useful firm and reliable landmark in the neck. ➢ The neck is divided into six Levels. The levels are identified by Roman numeral, increasing towards the chest. ➢ Level I: Submental and submandibular triangles. Ia is the submental triangle bound by the anterior bellies of the digastric and the mylohyoid. Ib

		is the triangle formed by the anterior and posterior bellies of the digastric and body of mandible. ➢ Level II: upper third including the upper jugular and jugulodigastric nodes and the upper posterior cervical nodes. Region bound by the digastric muscle superiorly and the hyoid bone (clinical landmark), or the carotid bifurcation (surgical landmark) inferiorly. IIa contains nodes in the region anterior to the spinal accessory nerve and IIb posterior to the nerve. ➢ Level III: middle third jugular nodes extending from the carotid bifurcation superiorly to the cricothyroid notch (clinical landmark), or inferior edge of cricoid cartilage (radiological landmark), or omohyoid muscle (surgical landmark). ➢ Level IV: lower jugular nodes extending from the omohyoid muscle superiorly to the clavicle inferiorly.

		➢ Level V: posterior triangle group of lymph nodes located along the lower half of the spinal accessory nerve and the transverse cervical artery. The supraclavicular nodes are also included in this group. The posterior boundary is the anterior border of the trapezius muscle, the anterior boundary is the posterior border of the sternocleidomastoid muscle, and the inferior boundary is the clavicle. ➢ Level VI: anterior compartment group comprises lymph nodes surrounding the midline visceral structures of the neck extending from the level of the hyoid bone superiorly to the suprasternal notch inferiorly. On each side, the lateral boundary is the medial border of the carotid sheath. Located within this compartment are the perithyroidal lymph nodes, paratracheal lymph nodes, lymph nodes along the recurrent laryngeal nerves, and

		precricoid lymph nodes.
26	E	Radical neck dissections ➢ Involves removal of all the ipsilateral lymph nodes from level I–V as well as the sternocleidomastoid muscle (SCM), spinal accessory nerve (SAN) and internal jugular vein (IJV). It does not include removal of the suboccipital nodes, periparotid nodes except for intraparotid nodes located in the posterior aspect of the submandibular triangle, buccal nodes, retropharyngeal nodes, or paratracheal nodes. ➢ If the ipsilateral cervical lymph nodes are resected but one or more of the non-lymphatic structures is preserved than it is known as a modified radical neck dissection (MRND). Type I MRND preserves the SAN, type II MRND preserves the SAN and IJV, and type III MRND preserves the SAN, IJV, and SCM. The type III MRND is also referred to as the 'functional neck dissection' ➢ Selective Neck Dissection (SND) involves cervical lymphadenectomy with preservation of one or more lymph node groups that are routinely removed in a RND. Thus for oral cavity cancers, SND (I–III) is commonly performed. For oropharyngeal,

		hypopharyngeal and laryngeal cancers, SND (II–IV) is the procedure of choice. ➢ Extended Neck Dissection—This refers to removal of one or more additional lymph node groups or non-lymphatic structures, or both, not encompassed by the RND.
27	J	Selective neck dissection II,III,IV, VI
28	A	Bilateral neck dissection ➢ Supraglottic carcinoma has occult metastases to cervical lymph nodes in up to 30% of cases (levels II–IV). They are bilateral in up to 20% due to a rich blood supply. Therefore when treating these cancers, apart from treating the primary tumour, the neck has to be considered as well. ➢ This can be managed by radiotherapy or surgery depending on the stage of the tumour, the patient preference and patient compliance. ➢ Metastatic neck disease is the most important factor in the spread of head and neck SCC from primary sites. The most commonly involved primary sites are the mucosal areas of the larynx, oropharynx, hypopharynx, and oral cavity. ➢ Lymph node (LN) metastasis reduces the survival rate of patients with SCC

		by half. The survival rate is less than 5% in patients who previously underwent surgery and have a recurrent metastasis in the neck. Therefore, control of the neck is one of the most important aspects in the successful management of these particular tumors.
29	E	Gwynne Evans dissector
30	M	Trousseau tracheal dilators
31	K	Transoral laser ➢ This can be treated with radiotherapy or transoral laser. However, if it is a pedunculated mass and complete surgical excision can be completed easily then transoral laser should be the preferred option. ➢ Transoral laser microsurgery is a form of minimally invasive surgery used to remove small and medium tumour and occasionally used for larger tumours. Transoral laser microsurgery allows access to tumours that are not reachable with robotic surgery. This technique helps to give as much speech and swallowing function as possible after surgery. ➢ T1 and T2 laryngeal squamous cell carcinoma is traditionally treated with radiotherapy. However, with the

		advent of trans-oral laser simple pedunculated masses can be excised with good cure rates and minimal morbidity.. ➢ Radiotherapy for laryngeal cancer is best given using three-dimensional conformal radiation therapy (3D-CRT). Conformal radiotherapy uses the same radiotherapy machine as normal radiotherapy treatment. However, a device called a multi-leaf collimator is used to arrange the shape of the beams so that they 'conform' to the area of the cancer. This ensures that a higher dose of radiation is given to the tumour. Healthy surrounding cells and nearby structures receive a lower dose of radiation, so the possibility of side effects is reduced. ➢ Intensity-modulated radiotherapy (IMRT) is a new type of radiotherapy that is able to shape treatment beams more precisely than 3D-CRT. This allows the dose of radiotherapy to be changed in different parts of the larynx and surrounding tissues. This can reduce the side effects of treatment.
32	H	Surveillance ➢ If this patient continues to smoke his dysplasia will become carcinoma *in situ*

		which can then become invasive carcinoma. Therefore, careful surveillance with regular biopsies is recommended. ➢ The core functions of cancer surveillance are the measurement of cancer incidence, morbidity, survival, and mortality for persons with cancer. It also includes the assessment of genetic predisposition, environmental and behavioural risk factors, screening practices, and the quality of care from prevention through palliation. ➢ Cancer surveillance tells us where we are in the effort to reduce the cancer burden and also generates the observations that form the basis for cancer research and interventions for cancer prevention and control.
33	I	Total laryngectomy ➢ Treatment for T4 squamous cell carcinoma is total laryngectomy accompanied by selective lateral neck dissection. Post operative radiotherapy provides further local control. ➢ This may also apply to T3 lesions; the alternative to surgery is chemoradiotherapy. ➢ Voice functions are generally replaced with voice prosthesis placed in the

		tracheoesophageal puncture created by the surgeon. The voice prosthesis vibrates the esophagus in lieu of the larynx. ➢ A second method is the use of anelectrolarynx. An electrolarynx is an external device that is placed against the neck and creates vibration that the speaker then articulates. The sound has been characterized as mechanical and robotic. ➢ A third method is called esophageal speech. The speaker pushes air into the esophagus and then pushes it back up, articulating speech sounds to speak. This method is time-consuming and difficult to learn.
34	J	Tracheostomy ➢ Treatment for this cancer would normally involve radiotherapy. However, in an emergency situation an airway must be created. ➢ Performing a laryngectomy would be considered over treatment in someone who could have organ preservation with radiotherapy. ➢ Laser debulking would be a good option if the department had equipment and expertise. However, there is always post operative swelling

		that should be borne in mind. ➢ A low tracheostomy makes subsequent laryngectomy difficult whereas a high tracheostomy has risks of seeding the tumour. In an emergency situation tracheostomy under local anaesthetic is the most common management.
35	F	Hormonal rhinitis ➢ Nonallergic rhinitis has seven basic subclassifications, as follows: (1) infectious rhinitis, (2) vasomotor rhinitis, (3) occupational rhinitis, (4) hormonal rhinitis, (5) drug-induced rhinitis, (6) gustatory rhinitis, and (7) nonallergic rhinitis with eosinophilia syndrome (NARES). ➢ A thorough history and physical examination aid the clinician in identifying the etiology and help direct the appropriate therapeutic course. ➢ Oestrogen causes upregulation of histamine receptors and therefore leads to rhinitis in up to 20% of pregnant ladies. The risk is greatly increased by smoking. Hormonal rhinitis can also occur in patients with low thyroid function. Pregnant women usually have symptoms of severe nasal congestion occurring during their second month of pregnancy, and this

		can persist until the baby is born. Symptoms typically disappear shortly after delivery.
36	I	Non-allergic occupational rhinitis ➢ Occupational Rhinitis may be defined as 'an inflammatory condition of the nose, which is characterized by intermittent or persistent symptoms (i.e. nasal congestion, sneezing, rhinorrhea, itching) and/or variable nasal airflow limitation and/or hypersecretion, due to causes and conditions attributable to a particular work environment and not to stimuli encountered outside the workplace'. ➢ Occupational rhinitis is different from work-exacerbated rhinitis (WER), which is pre-existing or concurrent (allergic or nonallergic) rhinitis that is worsened by, but not caused by, workplace exposures OR can develop in response to allergens, inhaled irritants, or corrosive gases. ➢ Generally non-allergic rhinitis is a medical condition of unknown cause, leading to symptoms very similar to allergic rhinitis, or hay-fever. Unlike allergies, which can be a seasonal problem, symptoms of non-allergic rhinitis are typically year-round.

		➢ Non-allergic rhinitis has many different forms: Vasomotor rhinitis is triggered by physical conditions such as strong odors, perfumes, changes in temperature and humidity, smoke, fumes and bright sunlight. Most patients experience a runny nose, post nasal drip and/or nasal congestion. Itching of the nose and eyes is typically not present. ➢ Infectious rhinitis is typically related to a viral or bacterial infection, and symptoms can mimic a sinus infection, with facial pain and green nasal discharge. However, these patients do not have evidence of a sinus infection on X-rays. This disease process resolves on its own within a few days, and responds to oral antibiotics in severe or prolonged cases, just as a sinus infection would.
37	D	Drug induced rhinitis ➢ Rhinitis is characterized by inflammation of the mucous membranes lining the nose and can be divided into two categories, allergic and non-allergic. ➢ Drug-induced is a type of non-allergic rhinitis. NSAIDS, β-blockers and ACE inhibitors can all lead to drug induced

		rhinitis. Whereas sensitivity to aspirin is more likely to cause rhinitis, beta-blocker and ACE inhibitors causes nasal blockage. When possible, the offending medication should be discontinued or substituted. ➢ Although there are no established treatment recommendations for drug-induced rhinitis other than avoidance, clinical experience suggests that it would be reasonable to initiate use of an intranasal corticosteroid spray to treat symptomatically. The addition of an intranasal antihistamine in combination with use of an intranasal corticosteroid may be considered as step-up therapy if the intranasal corticosteroid alone is not effective.
38	B	Atrophic rhinitis ➢ Granulomatous conditions lead to destruction of the nasal mucosa and turbinate bone allowing for larger airways. Paradoxically, the patient complains of nasal blockage, cacosmia and crusting. ➢ In atrophic rhinitis, the nasal cavities become roomy and are filled with foul smelling crusts which are black or dark green and dry, making expiration painful and difficult.

		➢ Microorganisms are known to multiply and produce a foul smell from the nose, though the patients may not be aware of this, because their elements (responsible for the perception of smell) have become atrophied. ➢ Patients usually complain of nasal obstruction despite the roomy nasal cavity, which can be caused either by the obstruction produced by the discharge in the nose, or as a result of sensory loss due to atrophy of nerves in the nose, so the patient is unaware of the air flow. In the case of the second cause, the sensation of obstruction is subjective. ➢ Bleeding from the nose may occur when the dried discharge are removed. Septal perforation and dermatitis of nasal vestibule can occur. The nose may show a saddle-nose deformity. ➢ Atrophic rhinitis is also associated with similar atrophic changes in the pharynx or larynx, producing symptoms pertaining to these structures. ➢ Hearing impairment can occur due to eustachian tube blockage causing middle ear effusion. ➢ Permanent loss of smell and impairment of taste may also be a

		result of this disease, even after the symptoms are cured.
39	A	Allergic rhinitis ➢ Allergic rhinitis occurs when an allergen, such as pollen, dust or animal dander is inhaled by an individual with a sensitized immune system. In such individuals, the allergen triggers the production of the antibody immunoglobulin E (IgE), which binds to mast cells and basophils containing histamine. ➢ IgE bound to mast cells are stimulated by pollen and dust, causing the release of inflammatory mediators such as histamine (and other chemicals. This usually causes sneezing, itchy and watery eyes, swelling and inflammation of the nasal passages, and an increase in mucus production. ➢ Symptoms vary in severity between individuals. Very sensitive individuals can experience hives or other rashes. ➢ Particulate matter in polluted air, and chemicals such as chlorine and detergents, which can normally be tolerated, can greatly aggravate allergic rhinitis. The commonest allergen is house dust mites' faeces.
40	D	Ethmoid infundibulum

		➢ The infundibulum is a funnel shaped 3-dimensional space that lies between the uncinate and the lamina papyracea. It allows passage of anterior ethmoid and maxillary sinus pathways. Depending on the superior attachment of the uncinate it may also contain frontal sinus drainage pathways. ➢ The infundibulum leads to a 2-dimensional gap between the uncinate and ethmoid bulla called the hiatus semilunaris. The hiatus semilunaris is bounded inferiorly by the sharp concave margin of the uncinate process of the ethmoid bone, and leads into the infundibulum, bounded above by the bulla ethmoidalis and below by the lateral surface of the uncinate process of the ethmoid.
41	B	Anterior osteomeatal unit ➢ The osteomeatal unit consists of the infundibulum along with the frontal recess and the maxillary sinus ostium. It is posterolateral to the uncinate process. ➢ The ethmoidal infundibulum is the most frequently involved region in inflammatory sinus disease and lies lateral to the uncinate process and

		cannot be seen directly. ➢ The natural maxillary ostium lies behind the uncinate process and therefore any openings seen must be accessory ostia.
42	J	Uncinate process ➢ Embryologically the lateral nasal wall forms five ridges (lamella) that become important structures. The first ridge becomes the uncinate bone. The second becomes the bulla ethmoidalis. The third becomes the middle turbinate. The fourth is the superior turbinate and the fifth is the supreme turbinate. ➢ The uncinate process, projects downward and backward from this part of the labyrinth; it forms a small part of the medial wall of the maxillary sinus, and articulates with the ethmoidal process of the inferior nasal concha. Anteriorly it is attached to the lateral nasal wall whilst posteriorly it is free. Inferiorly it is attached to the inferior turbinate and superiorly it is most often attached to the lamina papyracea (occasionally to the skull base or middle turbinate).
43	C	T1 N1a ➢ Scoring system for prognosis of

		differentiated thyroid cancer include the TNM Staging -Tumor, node, metastasis. Remarkable about the TNM staging for (differentiated) thyroid carcinoma is that the scoring is different according to age. Other prognostic systems commonly used are: AGES -Age, Grade, Extent of disease, Size AMES -Age, Metastasis, Extent of disease, Size MACIS -Metastasis, Age at presentation, Completeness of surgical resection, Invasion (extrathyroidal), Size (this is a modification of the AGES system). It is probably the most reliable staging method available.
44	D	T1 N1b
45	I	Recommend hearing aids. ➢ Otitis media with effusion is a common condition of early childhood. It is suggested there are associations with: prematurity, use of a pacifier, bottle feeding and parental smoking. Other congenital associations are cleft palate and conditions such as Down's syndrome. ➢ It is usual to instigate a period of observation for 3 months (with audiometry) and record the impact on development as over 50% of effusions resolve in that time frame.

		➢ Children with cleft palate and Down's syndrome require special consideration as effusions occur more commonly and at an early age. Children with Down's syndrome frequently have stenotic ear canals (40% of under 3s). They also suffer from frequent upper respiratory tract infections. Due to this combination insertion of grommets is more frequently associated with chronically discharging ears, which are far more difficult to manage. Therefore, NICE recommends in the first instance they should be fitted with hearing aids.
46	J	Repeat hearing test in 3 months ➢ Surgical management of glue ear requires there to be bilateral conductive hearing loss, proven over a minimum of 3 month period. Since the disease is fluctuating and self-limiting, a repeat of the hearing test should always be performed to avoid over treatment. ➢ Formal assessment of a child for otitis media should include a focused clinical history (listening, language, behaviour, milestones, infections: ear/respiratory), examination (otoscopy, development), hearing

		levels (tailored to developmental stage) and tympanometry. ➢ Current guidance stipulates hearing thresholds of 25–30 dBHL or worse averaged at 0.5, 1, 2 and 4 k Hz (in the better hearing ear) over 3 months should be considered for surgical intervention. ➢ Parents should be counselled as to the rationale behind observation and well as the likelihood of transient hearing loss which is self-limiting and has no adverse consequences.
47	J	Repeat hearing test in 3 months. ➢ As stated NICE only recommends surgical intervention for glue ear (otitis media with effusion) when the average hearing level in the better ear is 25–30 dBHL or worse. NICE does not recommend topical steroids/decongestants for the management of glue ear, although some people still try these despite no definitive evidence for there use. ➢ The good hearing ear will compensate for the loss on the opposite side. During the period of observation advice on educational and behavioural strategies to minimise the effects should be offered. However, these

		children are likely to develop otitis media with effusion that requires surgical intervention and therefore should be followed up. ➢ The presence of bilateral disease predicts a higher likelihood of more severe hearing loss and longer persistence and so should be considered for treatment.
48	E	Insert grommets and adenoidectomy. ➢ Once a decision has been taken to offer surgical intervention for OME in children, the insertion of ventilation tubes is recommended. By 12–18 months after intervention, no significant benefit in hearing levels has been demonstrated from surgery unless the ventilation tubes are still in place and functioning. ➢ Adjuvant adenoidectomy is not recommended in the absence of persistent and/or frequent upper respiratory tract symptoms. However this child has got frequent URTI and nasal blockage, hence adenoidectomy is indicated. ➢ Monopolar suction diathermy is commonly used to remove the adenoid under direct vision. The Trial for Alternative Regimens for Glue Ear

		Treatment (TARGET) showed benefit of adenoidectomy when the child suffers from glue ear +/-recurrent upper respiratory tract infections. ➢ It is recognised that there are some groups of children with OME who may benefit from early ventilation tube insertion. Examples are children requiring urgent surgery for airway impairment secondary to adenotonsillar hypertrophy and children with coexistent severe and profound hearing loss.
49	D	Insert grommets. ➢ Cleft palate results in impaired Eustachian tube function and renders children with cleft palate particularly susceptible to middle ear disease, particularly OME. ➢ Children with cleft palate and proven glue ear should be offered grommet insertions. However, prophylactic grommets should not be inserted after primary cleft closure. ➢ Careful audiology should be used to confirm the diagnosis before proceeding. All children with cleft palate should be managed by a multidisciplinary group which includes local professionals and the core cleft

		palate team. The sharing of care between these groups should be arranged to maximise the benefit to individual patients. ➢ Ventilation tube insertion has been shown to improve hearing in children with cleft palate but surgically treated children are more likely than the general population to require multiple operations with their attendant complications.
50	E	Fluticasone furoate ➢ It is important to know the underlying constituents of the most commonly prescribed ENT medications in the UK. ➢ Avamys (fluticasone furoate) is an intranasal steroid, similar to Nasonex and Flixonase. It also contains glucose anhydrous, dispersible cellulose, polysorbate 80, benzalkonium, disodium edentate and purified water. The delivery systems of these sprays vary slightly which is why a variety of preparations exist. ➢ It is a corticosteroid, but can be used long term as the systemic dose is considered negligible. The recommended dosage is two sprays in each nostril once a day (occasionally twice a day) each spray delivers

		approximately 27.5 micrograms of fluticasone furoate. This is not true for preparations such as Betnesol drops that can provide a systemic dose of steroid equivalent to around 3 mg of prednisolone
51	K	Ipratropium bromide. ➢ Rinatec can be used for rhinorrhoea as it is an antimuscarinic or anticholinergic. It implemented in cases of both allergic and non-allergic rhinosinusitis. ➢ It exerts its effects by the blockade of muscarinic acetylcholine receptors without specificity for subtypes and therefore inhibits degradation of cyclic guanosine monophosphate (cGMP). The result is an intracellular increase of cGMP concentration. Most likely due to actions of cGMP on intracellular calcium, this results in decreased mucus secretion. ➢ When used for by the respiratory physicians for conditions effecting lungs it affects the contractility of smooth muscle in the lung inhibiting bronchoconstriction. It does not diffuse into the blood, which prevents systemic side effects. Local side effects include dryness, irritation and

		epistaxis. Each metered dose is said to provide 21 μg of ipratropium bromide.
52	J	Iodoform, Benzoin & Storax ➢ Whitehead varnish is a powerful antiseptic substance that can be impregnated onto ribbon gauze and inserted into nasal or oral cavities after surgery. It is comprised of iodoform 10 g, benzoin 10 g, prepared storax 7.5 g, Balsam of Tolu 5 g and solvent mixed to 100 mL. ➢ It remains sterile in regions of high bacterial load. The aromatic resins are slowly broken down to produce benzoic acid, which is a potent antiseptic. It has been used for over 100 years and is attributed to Walter Whitehead who became a fellow of the Royal College of Surgeons of Edinburgh in 1866. It remains a well utilised substance in the realms of ear, nose and throat surgery.
53	B	Salivary lesions ➢ The parapharyngeal space is a potential inverted pyramidal space extending from the skull base to the greater horn of the hyoid bone. It is divided into two compartments (pre- and post-styloid) by the tensor veli palatine muscle and fascia, which

		extends from the styloid process to the fascia covering the muscle and crosses posterior into the parapharyngeal fat. ➢ The majority of lesions in the pre-styloid parapharyngeal space are salivary neoplasms, of which the most common is pleomorphic adenoma. They may originate from the deep lobe parotid gland, minor salivary glands or from ectopic salivary cell formation. The other lesions reported in the pre-styloid space include lipomas and neurogenic tumours. ➢ In general parapharyngeal space tumours present with subtle signs and symptoms and grow slowly. Symptoms do not often appear until the lesion is greater than 2.5 cm in size, which then has a mass effect. ➢ Sinister signs include pain, cranial nerve palsies and trismus. Palpitations, headaches, hypertension tremor and flushing may indicate the presence of catecholamine excess from a paraganglioma within the parapharyngeal space. ➢ The majority of neoplasms in the parapharyngeal space present as an asymptotic neck or oropharyngeal mass caused medial displacement of

		the lateral pharyngeal wall, ipsilateral tonsil and/or soft palate. ➢ Infection in the pre-styloid compartment usually causes fever, chills, and neck pain and trismus as well as anterolateral displacement of the ipsilateral palatine tonsil.
54	C	Neurogenic lesions ➢ These lesions occur more commonly in the post-styloid space and represents 20–30% of tumours in this area. The tumours arise from the neural structures of the lower cranial nerves, sympathetic chain and paraganglia are the source for schwannomas, paragangliomas and neurofibromas. ➢ Other tumours of the parapharyngeal space include lymphoreticular and metastatic lesions. Metastasise from thyroid carcinoma and sarcoma may first present in the parapharyngeal space. ➢ Overall, neoplasms of the parapharyngeal space represent 0.5% of all head and neck tumours. They maybe divided into primary lesions with originate form the *in situ* structures, tumours that invade the area by extension from adjacent spaces and metastatic lesions.

		➢ However the majority (80%) are benign lesions mainly affecting adults. Children tend to get parapharyngeal infections arising from pharyngitis, tonsillitis, otitis, mastoiditis, parotiditis and cervical lymphadenitis. Odontogenic infections also contribute by way of indirect spread from adjacent deep neck spaces. ➢ In contrast to infection in the pre-styloid compartment, infection in the post-styloid space is associated with little or no pain, trismus, or obvious swelling. However, spread to the carotid sheath may result in Lemierre's syndrome, consisting of internal jugular vein thrombosis or carotid artery aneurysm or rupture, ipsilateral Horner's syndrome and cranial nerve palsies (IX–XII).
55	L	Pleomorphic adenoma ➢ A pleomorphic adenoma is mixed benign tumour may arise in any of the salivary glands but most commonly in the parotid gland. It is a true adenoma showing pseudomesenchymal differentiation with foci of mucus, hyaline and cartilage thought to be derived from the intercalated duct cells and myoepithelium.

- Microscopic examination reveals solid strands of cuboidal and cylindrical epithelial cells having stellate processes or cells with halos that resemble cartilage cells.
- Although it is classified as a benign tumour, pleomorphic adenomas have the capacity to grow to large proportions and may undergo malignant transformation, to form carcinoma ex-pleomorphic adenoma, a risk that increases with time.
- The diagnosis of salivary gland tumors utilizes both tissue sampling(FNAC and Core biopsy) and radiographic studies like ultrasound, computer tomography (CT) and magnetic resonance imaging (MRI).
- Fine needle aspiration biopsy (FNA), operated in experienced hands, can determine whether the tumor is malignant in nature with sensitivity around 90%. FNA can also distinguish primary salivary tumor from metastatic disease.
- Overall, the mainstay of the treatment for salivary gland tumor is surgical resection. Surgical treatment of parotid gland tumours may be difficult because of the anatomical relationship of the

		facial nerve. There is a trend now to use a modified face lift incision to remove parotid lesion.
	N	Salivary mucocele ➢ This refers to a mucous cyst of the oral mucosa due to mucus extravasation. The mucocele has a bluish translucent color, and is more commonly found in children and young adults. ➢ The most common location to find a mucocele is the surface of the lower lip. It can also be found on the inner side of the cheek on the anterior ventral tongue, and the floor of the mouth. When found on the floor of the mouth, the mucocele is referred to as a ranula. They are rarely found on the upper lip. ➢ A variant of a mucocele is found on the palate, retromolar pad, and posterior buccal mucosa. Known as a 'superficial mucocele', this type presents as single or multiple vesicles and bursts into an ulcer. Despite healing after a few days, superficial mucoceles recur often in the same location. ➢ Microscopically, mucoceles appears as granulation tissue surrounding mucin. Since inflammation occurs concurrently, neutrophils and foamy

		histiocytes usually are present. Some mucoceles spontaneously resolve of their own accord after a short time. Others are chronic and require surgical removal. Recurrence may occur, and thus the adjacent salivary gland is excised as a preventive measure. ➢ Several types of procedures are available for the surgical removal of mucoceles. These include laser and minimally-invasive techniques which means recovery times are reduced drastically. ➢ A non-surgical option that may be effective for a small or newly identified mucocele is to rinse the mouth thoroughly with salt water four to six times a day for a few days. This may draw out the fluid trapped underneath the skin without further damaging the surrounding tissue.
57	D	Adenolymphoma (Warthin's tumour) ➢ This is a benign tumour that occurs almost exclusively in the parotid gland of elderly men. The incidence of bilateral lesions is about 10% but rarely synchronously. ➢ Macroscopically, the sectioned surface is finely cystic. Microscopically, there are cystic spaces lined by a double

layer of epithelium with eosinophilic cytoplasm. Warthin's tumours characteristically have lymphoid tissue lying between microscopic cysts.

- Warthin's tumour is the second most common benign parotid tumor and primarily affects older individuals (age 60–70 years). There is a slight female predilection according to recent studies, but historically it has been associated with a strong male predilection. This change s possibly due to the tumor's association with cigarette smoking and the growing use of cigarettes by women.
- The tumor is slow growing, painless, and usually appears in the tail of the parotid gland near the angle of the mandible. In 5–14% of cases, Warthin's tumor is bilateral, but the two masses usually are at different times. Warthin's tumor is highly unlikely to become malignant. The appearance of this tumor under the microscope is unique. There are cystic spaces surrounded by two uniform rows of cells with centrally placed pyknotic nuclei. The cystic spaces have epithelium referred to as papillary infoldings that protrude into them.

		Additionally, the epithelium has lymphoid stroma with germinal center formation. ➢ The differential diagnosis includes sebaceous lymphadenoma and oncocytoma. Most of these tumors are treated with surgical removal. It is non recurrent.
58	C	Adenoid cystic carcinoma. ➢ This is the second most common malignant salivary gland tumour and tends to spread along nerve sheath leading to facial pain and sometimes nerve palsy. The incidence of lymph node metastasis is low and distance metastases to the lung are rare. ➢ Histologically it shows a Swiss cheese pattern with adenoid cellular structures having both small and large cystic spaces filled with mucus. The cysts develop from the accumulation of mucus secreted by epithelial cells which are embedded in hyaline stroma. ➢ Adenoid cystic cancer (AdCC) is a rare type of cancer that can exist in many different body sites. It most often occurs in the areas of the head and neck, in particular the salivary glands. AdCC represents 28% of malignant

		submandibular gland tumors, making it the single most common malignant salivary gland tumor in this region. ➢ Patients may survive for years with metastases because this tumor is generally well-differentiated and slow growing. ➢ Primary treatment for this cancer is surgical removal with clean margins. This surgery can prove challenging in the head and neck region due to this tumour's tendency spread along nerve tracts. Adjuvant or palliative radiotherapy is commonly given following surgery. In some cases surgery is not a reasonable option, however radiation used alone may provide an effective treatment. Chemotherapy is used for metastatic disease. Chemotherapy is considered on a case by case basis, as there is limited trial data on the positive effects of chemotherapy.
59	J	Mucoepidermoid carcinoma ➢ Mucoepidermoid carcinoma may arise in any salivary gland tissue, but mainly seen in the parotid gland. The lesion can also be found in other organs such as bronchi, lacrimal sac and thyroid. ➢ It is the commonest malignant salivary

		gland tumour; haemangiomas are the commonest benign parotid tumour in children. Mucoepidermoid carcinoma occurs in adults, with peak incidence from 20–40 years of age. It presents as painless, slow-growing mass that is firm or hard. The tumour is not encapsulated and is characterized by squamous cells, mucus-secreting cells, and intermediate cells. ➢ They are classified histologically into low grade, intermediate and high grade. The low grade tumours exhibit a benign behaviour and a good prognosis, whilst the other two grades are more aggressive. The high grade (or undifferentiated) mucoepidermoid lesions metastasise early and carry a poor prognosis. However, the clinical progression is not always accurately predicted by the histological appearance. ➢ Recently, a causal link with cytomegalovirus (CMV) has been strongly implicated.
60	J	Upper airways resistance syndrome ➢ This is milder variant of obstructive sleep apnoea. Symptoms are the same, however, sleep study fails to reveal any apnoea/hypopnoea. There are

			however, frequent arousals from sleep. It is thought the increase work of the respiratory muscles to open an obstructed airways leads to arousal, and hence disruption of sleep cycle and failure to thrive. ➢ Upper Airway Resistance Syndrome or UARS is a sleep disorder characterized by airway resistance to breathing during sleep. Polysomnography (sleep study) with the use of a probe to measure Pes (esophageal pressure) is the gold standard diagnostic test for UARS. Apneas and hypopneas are absent or present in low numbers. Multiple snore arousals may be seen, and if an esophageal probe (Pes) is used, progressive elevation of esophageal pressure fluctuations terminating in arousals is noted. ➢ UARS can also be diagnosed using a nasal cannula/pressure transducer to measure the inspiratory airflow vs time signal. During sleep the muscles of the airway become relaxed. The relaxation of these muscles in turn reduces the diameter of the airway. Typically, the airway of a UARS patient is already restricted or reduced in size, and this natural relaxation reduces the airway

			further. Therefore, breathing becomes labored. It can be likened to breathing through a coffee straw. ➢ Pathophysiology of UARS is similar to obstructive sleep apnea / hypopnea syndrome in that abnormal airway resistance in the upper airway during sleep leads to unwanted physiologic consequences. Increased upper airway resistance in this disorder does not lead to cessation of airflow (apnea) or decrease in airflow (hypopnea), but instead leads to an arousal secondary to increased work of breathing to overcome the resistance. Repeated and multiple arousals (which the patient is usually unaware of) result in an abnormal sleep architecture and daytime somnolence (sleepiness). Arousals result in sympathetic activation, and UARS is therefore likely to cause hypertension similar to obstructive sleep apnea syndrome (This has not been verified in large clinical populations because of the relatively small number of patients with UARS in the larger epidemiologic studies so far). ➢ Treatment is with CPAP and is similar to that in obstructive sleep apnoea

61	I	Periodic limb movement disorder ➢ This is a condition where the early phases of sleep are unable to block motor instructions from the motor cortex. This leads to periodic leg movement and therefore arousal. This disease probably has a similar aetiology to restless leg syndrome. ➢ Patients with periodic limb movement disorder complain of excessive daytime sleepiness (Eds), falling asleep during the day, trouble falling asleep at night, and difficulty staying asleep throughout the night. Patients also display involuntary limb movements that occur at periodic intervals anywhere from 20–40 sec apart. They often only last the first half of the night during non-REM sleep stages. Movements do not occur during REM because of muscle atonia. ➢ Periodic limb movement disorder is often treated with anti-Parkinson's medication. These include anticonvulsants, benzodiazepines, and narcotics. Patients must stay on these medications in order to experience relief for there is no known cure for this disorder. It is also advised to not consume caffeine, alcohol or

		antidepressants as these substances could worsen the PLMD symptoms. ➢ Other medications aimed at reducing or eliminating the leg jerks or the arousals can be prescribed. Non-ergot derived dopaminergic drugs (pramipexole and ropinirole) are preferred. Other dopaminergic agents such as co-careldopa, co-beneldopa, pergolide, or lisuride may also be used. These drugs decrease or eliminate both the leg jerks and the arousals. These medications are also successful for the treatment of restless legs syndrome.
62	C	Idiopathic hypersomnolence ➢ This should only be considered when all other diagnoses have been ruled out. It tends to affect pubescent boys who have difficulty waking up and sleep for long periods but do not feel refreshed. They require frequent daytime naps. Polysomnography is normal. At its extreme it can be part of a hyperphagia-hypersomnolence syndrome called Klein–Levin syndrome. ➢ Like narcolepsy, idiopathic hypersomnolence is a condition characterised by excessive sleepiness. Patients also experience difficulty in waking (either in the morning or at the

		end of nap periods during the day). As with narcolepsy, patients with this condition often sleep for long periods but, unlike patients with narcolepsy, in whom sleep attacks can occur anytime without warning, patience with idiopathic hypersomnolence have a greater degree of control over their sleep, and do not suffer from cataplexy or the other features of the full narcolepsy syndrome, such as sleep paralysis, hallucinations and automatisms. ➢ Although about 25% of patients experience spontaneous improvement in their condition, it can be life-long and can require treatment with similar stimulant medications to those which are used for treating narcolepsy. Treatment usually involves the use of medication to counter daytime sleepiness and lifestyle changes. Excessive daytime tiredness is usually treated by medicines that stimulate the central nervous system, including amphetamine, methamphetamine, methylphenidate and modafinil.
63	A	Central sleep apnoea ➢ This occurs when the brain does not send signals to the respiratory

			apparatus to inspire during sleep. This causes hypoxaemia and hypercapnia leading to eventual arousal. ➢ Polysomnography shows apnoea with failed respiratory effort. In pure central sleep apnea the brain's respiratory control centres are imbalanced during sleep. Blood levels of carbon dioxide, and the neurological feedback mechanism that monitors them, do not react quickly enough to maintain an even respiratory rate, with the entire system cycling between apnea and hyperpnea, even during wakefulness. There is no effort made to breathe during the pause in breathing: there are no chest movements and no struggling. After the episode of apnea, breathing may be faster (hyperpnea) for a period of time; a compensatory mechanism to blow off retained waste gases and absorbs more oxygen. ➢ In central sleep apnea, the basic neurological controls for breathing rate malfunction and fail to give the signal to inhale, causing the individual to miss one or more cycles of breathing. If the pause in breathing is long enough, the percentage of oxygen in the circulation will drop to a lower than normal level

		and the concentration of carbon dioxide will build to a higher than normal level. In turn, these conditions of hypoxia and hypercapnia will trigger additional effects on the body. The exact effects of the condition will depend on how severe the apnea is and on the individual characteristics of the person having the apnea.
64	E	Narcolepsy ➢ This is a sleep disorder characterised by excessive daytime somnolence. It starts in early adulthood. Patients often require frequent daytime naps which can occur involuntarily. They complain hallucinations going to sleep and waking up. ➢ Treatment is tailored to the individual, based on symptoms and therapeutic response. The time required to achieve optimal control of symptoms is highly variable, and may take several months or longer. Medication adjustments are frequently necessary, and complete control of symptoms is seldom possible. While oral medications are the mainstay of formal narcolepsy treatment, lifestyle changes are also important. ➢ The main treatment of excessive

		daytime sleepiness in narcolepsy is central nervous system stimulants such as methylphenidate, amphetamine, methamphetamine, modafinil (Provigil), a new stimulant with a different pharmacologic mechanism, and/or armodafinil (Nuvigil). Other medications used are codeine and selegiline. Another drug that is used is atomoxetine (Strattera), a non-stimulant and norepinephrine reuptake inhibitor (NRI), that has little or no abuse potential. ➢ In many cases, planned regular short naps can reduce the need for pharmacological treatment of the EDS but only improve symptoms for a short duration. A 120 minute nap provided benefit for 3 hours in patient alertness where as a 15 minute nap provided no benefit.
65	I	Subperiosteal abscess. ➢ Subperiosteal abscess should be suspected in cases of periorbital cellulitis that fail to improve on broad-spectrum intravenous antibiotics. ➢ Repeated clinical examinations are necessary to evaluate improvement or lack of improvement following intravenous antibiotic therapy and the

		need for surgical intervention.
66	H	Pre-septal cellulitis. ➢ The treatment should include a broad spectrum intravenous antibiotic, such as co-amoxiclav, and frequent review of vision as an inpatient. ➢ Most of current antibiotics are semisynthetic modifications of various natural compounds. These include, for example, the beta-lactam antibacterials, which include the penicillins (produced by fungi in the genus *Penicillium*), the cephalosporins, and the carbapenems. ➢ Compounds that are still isolated from living organisms are the aminoglycosides, whereas other antibacterials—for example, the sulfonamides, the quinolones, and the oxazolidinones—are produced solely by chemical synthesis. In accordance with this, many antibacterial compounds are classified on the basis of chemical/biosynthetic origin into natural, semisynthetic, and synthetic. ➢ Another classification system is based on biological activity; in this classification, antibacterials are divided into two broad groups according to their biological effect on

		microorganisms: bactericidal agents kill bacteria, and bacteriostatic agents slow down or stall bacterial growth.
67	G	Pott's Puffy tumour. ➢ Frontal sinusitis can lead to osteomyelitis and destruction of the anterior table, with subsequent dehiscence. This is known as Pott's Puffy tumour, first described by Sir Percivall Pott in 1760. Although it can affect all ages, it is mostly found among teenagers and adolescents. The infection can also spread inwards, leading to an intracranial abscess. ➢ This type of chronic osteomyelitis of the frontal bone is confused with acute sub-periosteal abscess of the frontal bone, which presents as a discrete collection over the frontal sinus. ➢ The most common cause is frontal sinusitis. Other causes include trauma, cocaine abuse and craniotomy (rare). ➢ Investigations should make sure the posterior table is intact. ➢ Surgery should be to gain microbiology sensitivities and better the underlying sinus disease if possible. However, full endoscopic drainage of the frontal sinus is difficult and can lead to scarring with ensuing complications.

		Open drainage can lead to a chronic fistula. Treatment generally consists of surgical drainage, and long-term (6–8 weeks) use of antibiotics.
68	B	Cavernous sinus thrombosis ➢ This is a dangerous complication of periorbital cellulitis with a high mortality. Fortunately, the incidence of cavernous sinus thrombosis has been decreased greatly with the advent of effective antimicrobial agents. ➢ Cavernous sinus thrombosis (CST) is the formation of a blood clot within the cavernous sinus, a cavity at the base of the brain which drains deoxygenated blood from the brain back to the heart. Because of its complex neurovascular anatomic relationship, cavernous sinus thrombosis is the most important of any intracranial septic thrombosis. ➢ *Staphylococcus aureus* and *Streptococcus* are often the causative bacteria. ➢ Cavernous sinus thrombosis symptoms include; decrease or loss of vision, chemosis, exophthalmos (bulging eyes), headaches, and paralysis of the cranial nerves which course through the cavernous sinus.

		➢ This infection is life-threatening and requires immediate treatment, which usually includes antibiotics and sometimes surgical drainage. Treatment with anticoagulants is still debated. Cavernous sinus thrombosis is usually a late complication of an infection of the central face or paranasal sinuses.
69	C	Cerebral abscess ➢ Intracranial abscesses are uncommon, serious, life-threatening infections. They include brain abscess and subdural or extradural empyema and are classified according to the anatomical location or the etiologic agent. ➢ The triad of fever, headache (often severe and on the side of the abscess), and focal neurologic deficit occurs in less than half of patients. Common symptoms and signs include: Headache, Mental status changes (may indicate cerebral edema), Focal neurologic deficits, Fever, Seizures, Nausea and vomiting, Nuchal rigidity, Papilloedema. ➢ A suddenly worsening headache, followed by emerging signs of meningismus, is often associated with

rupture of the abscess.

- The clinical manifestations of brain abscess are initially nonspecific, which can lead to delay in diagnosis. Brain abscess usually manifests as symptoms of a space-occupying lesion. The symptoms and signs include the following: Low-grade or high-grade fever, Persistent headache (often localized),Drowsiness, Confusion, Stupor, General or focal seizures, Nausea and vomiting, Focal motor or sensory impairments, Papilledema, Ataxia, Hemiparesis, Neck stiffness
- Investigations include:-
- CBC count with differential and platelet count, ESR and CRP
- Serological tests for some pathogens (eg, serum immunoglobulin G antibodies, CSF polymerase chain reaction [PCR] for *Toxoplasma*)
- Blood cultures (at least 2; preferably before antibiotic usage)
- Cerebrospinal fluid analysis
- Abscess aspirate (obtained via stereotactic CT or surgery)
- CT scanning, preferably with contrast administration, provides a rapid means of detecting the size, the number, and the location of abscesses, and it has

		become the mainstay of diagnosis and follow-up care. ➢ Many authorities consider MRI to be the first diagnostic method in the diagnosis of brain abscess. ➢ Treatment includes broad spectrum IV antibiotcs, IV Fluids and Drainage of abscess apart from treating the sinusitis
70	L	Sofradex ➢ Sofradex contains framycetin which is an antibiotic belonging to the aminoglycoside class. It has poor systemic absorption and is used in topical preparations for infections of the skin, nose, ears and eyes. ➢ Dexamethasone is a synthetic member of the glucocorticoid class of steroid drugs. It acts as an anti-inflammatory and immunosuppressant. It is about four times more potent than preditionisolone. ➢ Gramicidin is an antimicrobial cyclic polypeptide active in vitro against many gram positive bacteria. It is used for the local treatment of susceptible infections, sometimes in combination with other antimicrobial agents and frequently with a corticosteroid. ➢ In terms of pharmokinetic properties,

		framycetin Sulphate absorption occurs from inflamed skin and wounds. Once absorbed it is rapidly excreted by the kidneys in active form. It has been reported to have a half life of 2–3 hours Gramicidin has properties similar to those of Tyrothricin and is too toxic to be administered systemically. Dexamethasone is readily absorbed from the gastro-intestinal tract. It has a biological half-life in plasma of about 190 min.
71	K	Otosporin - Otosporin is a topical ear drops containing polymyxin B sulphate, neomycin sulphate, hydrocortisone EP. Neomycin is similar to other aminoglycosides and has excellent activity against gram negative bacteria, and has partial activity against gram positive bacteria. It is the most cochleotoxic aminoglycoside. - Otosporin solution is a bactericidal preparation active against all the pathogens commonly found in bacterial infections of the ear. - Neomycin sulphate is bactericidal against a wide range of gram positive and negative bacterial pathogens including *staphylococci, streptococci,*

		Escherichia, Enterobacter, Klebsiella, Haemophilus, Proteus, Salmonella and *Shigella* species. It is also active against some strains of the *pseudomonas aeruginosa* and against *mycobacterium tuberculosis* and *Neisseria gonorrhoea*. Neomycin exerts its bactericidal effect by interfering with the protein synthesis of susceptible organisms. ➢ Polymyxin B is bactericidal against a wide range of gram negative bacilli including *Pseudomonas* spp., *Escherichia coli, Enterobacter* spp., *Klebsiella* spp., and *Haemophilus influenzae*. It exerts a bactericidal effect by binding to acid phospholipids in the cell wall and membranes of the bacterium, thereby rendering ineffective the osmotic barrier normally provided by the cell membrane. This leads to escape of the cell contents and the death of the organism. Polymyxin B is an antibiotic primarily used for resistant gram-negative infections. It is derived from the bacterium *Bacillus polymyxa*.
72	J	Otomize ➢ Otomize ear spray contains 0.1% dexamethasone, 3250 units/mL neomycin sulphate and 2% glacial

		acetic acid. ➢ A solution of 2% acetic acid acts as an antifungal and antibacterial agent in the external ear canal. It may be used to treat mild otitis externa but severe cases require an anti-inflammatory preparation with or without an anti-infective drug. Neomycin is a member of the aminoglycoside family of antibiotics. It is used to treat infections caused by a wide variety of bacteria. Neomycin works by interfering with the production of proteins that are essential for the bacteria's survival. It binds to components in bacterial cells, making the bacteria produce abnormal proteins that can't perform their normal function. The production of these abnormal proteins ultimately kills the bacteria and this clears up the infection. Glacial acetic acid is included in this spray to produce an acid environment in the ear which is unfavourable for bacteria to survive in. This helps control any infection. ➢ The combination of the three medicines in Otomize ear spray is used to treat infection and inflammation of the outer ear. The spray is administered directly into the ear

		opening to produce a local effect in the outer ear canal.
73	H	Locorten Vioform ➢ Locorten Vioform is topical ear drop containing Flumethasone (a corticosteroid) and Clioquinol (Iodochlorhydroxyquin) an anti-fungal drug and antiprotozoal drug. ➢ It may be used to treat otitis externa. It is contraindicated if there is hypersensitivity to any component of the formulation or iodine, perforation of the tympanic membrane and in children under 2-years-old. Long-term continuous topical therapy should be avoided since this can lead to adrenal suppression. ➢ Topical application of clioquinol-containing preparations may lead to a marked increase in protein-bound iodine (PBI). The results of thyroid function tests, such as PBI, radioactive iodine and butanol extractable iodine, may be affected. However, other thyroid function tests, such as the T3 resin sponge test or T4 determination, are unaffected. ➢ Locorten Vioform is generally well tolerated, but may cause burning, itching or a rash. Very occasionally it

		may cause hair discolouration.
74	D	Canesten ➢ Canesten contains clotrimazole which is an antifungal medication commonly used in the treatment of fungal infections. It is available as an over-the-counter substance in various dosage forms, e.g. drops or cream. It is also available as a troche or throat lozenge (prescription only). ➢ For ear infection, it is often applied in liquid form, as ear drops. Otomycosis can be slow to eradicate because of spores, so the usual course for an anti-fungal agent is approximately 4 weeks. Clotrimazole is also commonly found in conjunction with the steroid betamethasone for its anti-inflammatory properties. ➢ Interestingly, Clotrimazole is also used to treat the sickling of cells in patients with sickle cell anemia by blocking ion channels in the red blood cell membrane, keeping ions and water within the cell. However, the primary mechanism of action of clotrimazole is against the division and growing of fungi. Clotrimazole alters the permeability of the fungal cell wall and inhibits the activity of enzymes within

		the cell. Studies show that minimal concentrations of clotrimazole causes leakage of intracellular phosphorus compounds into the ambient medium along with the breakdown of cellular nucleic acids and an accelerated k+ efflux which subsequently leads to the cell's death.
75	H	Oesophageal foreign body ➢ The sudden onset of dysphagia after a meal suggests an impacted foreign body, which may be food or denture in the elderly population. In children, ingestion of coin is a common problem. ➢ Ingested foreign body usually passes through the alimentary canal without any complication but occasionally they may become lodged in the lumen of the oesophagus. The object commonly becomes impacted in the cervical oesophagus at the level or just below cricopharyngeus. ➢ Few foreign bodies may perforate the oesophagus and even fewer may migrate extraluminally and be misdiagnosed as asthma. Blunt objects, like a coin, may cause perforation of the oesophagus by a mechanism involving time, pressure and foreign body reaction, which allows erosion of

		the oesophageal wall. To avoid such complication, it is important to identify and remove any 'hard' foreign body from the oesophagus as soon as possible.
76	C	Globus pharyngeus ➢ Globus pharyngeus describes the sensation of a lump or foreign body sensation in the throat for which clinical examination does not reveal any cause. It is most common in females in the fifth decade. ➢ Proposed aetiological theories include laryngopharyngeal acid reflux or a disorder of pharyngeal and/or oesophageal motility. ➢ Pharyngeal measurements of pH are generally normal, raising the possibility that acid may trigger vagally-mediated cricopharyngeal muscle spasm rather than the direct effect of acid on the pharynx. Motor dysfunction has been demonstrated in some patients including raised cricopharyngeal sphincter pressure, mid-oesophageal dysmotility and poor lower oesophageal relaxation, although debate ensures as to whether these are primary phenomena or secondary to acid.

		➢ There is no good evidence that thyroid nodules or enlargement are associated with globus. ➢ The strongest associated factors are undoubtedly anxiety, stress and other forms of psychological distress. Unfortunately these factors increase cricopharyngeal muscle spasm, which leads to worse symptoms of globus and heightened anxiety about the condition. ➢ The vicious cycle can therefore be self-perpetuating, and can only be broken by firm reassurance often by an ENT specialist who can confirm a normal examination on flexible nasendoscopy.
77	G	Oesophageal candidiasis. ➢ The history of drug addiction raises the possibility of a coexistent infection such as HIV associated with a degree of immunodeficiency, which in turn may give rise to candidiasis. When occurring in the oesophagus, this can cause pain on swallowing and dysphagia as a result. ➢ Esophageal candidiasis is an opportunistic infection of the esophagus by Candida albicans. The disease occurs in patients in immunocompromised states, including

		post-chemotherapy and in AIDS. It is also known as candidal esophagitis or monilial esophagitis. ➢ Patients with esophageal candidiasis present with odynophagia, or painful swallowing. Longstanding esophageal candidiasis can result in weight loss. There is often concomitant thrush. Some patients present with esophageal candidiasis as a first presentation of systemic candidiasis. ➢ Patients where esophageal candidiasis is suspected should undergo esophagogastroduodenoscopy if it is safe to do so. Endoscopy often reveals classic diffuse raised plaques that characteristically can be removed from the mucosa by the endoscope. ➢ Brushing or biopsy of the plaques shows yeast and pseudohyphae that are characteristic of Candida species. ➢ The current first-line treatment is a single dose of fluconazole (750 mg). Other therapy options include: nystatin, other oral triazoles, such as itraconazole , caspofungin, used in refractory or systemic cases, amphotericin B, used in refractory or systemic cases.
78	E	Myasthenia gravis

			➢ A number of conditions may at first glance fit this rubric, however it is the worsening of dysphagia as the meal progresses which is suggestive of the progressive lethargy and tiring associated with myasthenia gravis. ➢ This condition is considered to be an autoimmune channelopathy with antibodies directed against the body's own proteins. ➢ There is a slight genetic predisposition: particular HLA types seem to predispose for MG (B8 and DR3 with DR1 more specific for ocular myasthenia). ➢ Up to 75% of patients have an abnormality of the thymus; 10% have a thymoma, a tumor (either benign or malignant) of the thymus, and other abnormalities are frequently found. The disease process generally remains stationary after thymectomy. ➢ The edrophonium test is infrequently performed to identify MG; its application is limited to the situation when other investigations do not yield a conclusive diagnosis. This test requires the intravenous administration of edrophonium chloride (Tensilon, Reversol) or

		neostigmine (Prostigmin), drugs that block the breakdown of acetylcholine by cholinesterase (cholinesterase inhibitors) and temporarily increases the levels of acetylcholine at the neuromuscular junction. In patients with myasthenia gravis involving the eye muscles, edrophonium chloride will briefly relieve weakness.
79	D	Ménière's disease ➢ The symptoms of tinnitus and hearing loss preceding the onset of vertigo lasting several hours are typical of Ménière's syndrome. ➢ Ménière's disease (MD) consists of a paroxysmal triad of vertigo, unilateral fluctuating hearing loss and tinnitus associated with a feeling of aural fullness. Therefore, true MD can only be diagnosed at *post*-mortem. ➢ Migraine associated vertigo can mimic MD in its presentation as the duration of vertigo can be similar, although severe headache is usually the most significant symptom. ➢ Treatment is with vestibular sedatives during acute attacks. Betahistidine (a vasodilator) and diuretics are used prophylactically but the evidence base is not strong. Reduction of dietary salt,

		caffeine smoking may be helpful. Residual hearing may need amplification. ➢ Persistent and severe cases may be treated by endolymphatic sac decompression, vestibular neuroectomy, labyrinthectomy (surgical or chemical with aminoglycoside injection through the middle ear).
80	C	Benign Paroxysmal Positional Vertigo (BPPV) ➢ The brief nature of the vertigo together with its predominance in a particular and reproducible direction is suggestive of BPPV. ➢ Whilst most cases of BPPV seen in an ENT clinic will be idiopathic, head injury is a recognised predisposing factor in its aetiology. This is the commonest cause of recurrent vertigo. It is caused by otoliths breaking away from the otoconia in the utricle or saccule and passing into the posterior semicircular canal. ➢ Movement of the head in certain positions causes the otolith to stimule of the vestibular organ. Two treatments have been found effective for relieving symptoms of posterior

		canal BPPV: the canalith repositioning procedure or Epley manoeuvre, and the liberatory or Semont manoeuver. ➢ Epley manoeuvre employs gravity to move the calcium build-up that causes the condition. The particle repositioning manoeuver can be performed during a clinic visit by health professionals or taught to patients to practice at home. ➢ In the Semont manoeuver, patients themselves are able to achieve canalith repositioning. Both treatments, when performed by a health professional, appear to be equally effective. The Epley manoeuver does not address the actual presence of the particles (otoconia), rather it changes their location where they do not cause these problems.
81	G	Psychogenic ➢ Wooziness implies non specific dizziness rather than true vertigo. Its presence within a shopping mall indicates that there may be an element of agoraphobia. Psychogenic dizziness is particularly common in females. ➢ Hyperventilation leads respiratory alkalosis and associated hypocalcemia which in turn causes the tingling

		sensation. ➢ The other differential is a panic attack. Psychogenic dizziness should not be confused with psychogenic fugue which is a rare psychiatric disorder characterized by reversible amnesia for personal identity, including the memories, personality and other identifying characteristics of individuality. The state is usually short-lived (ranging from hours to days), but can last months or longer. ➢ Dissociative fugue usually involves unplanned travel or wandering, and is sometimes accompanied by the establishment of a new identity.
82	B	Acute vestibular failure ➢ Sudden severe vertigo lasting for more than 24 hours and associated with vomiting is likely to be acute labyrinthitis causing vestibular failure. This condition may follow an upper respiratory tract infection and can be quite debilitating, usually rendering the patient bed bound for one to two days, but it can last for a couple of weeks with gradual improvement. Central compensation takes place during the recovery period. ➢ Acute labyrinthitis is thought to be due

		to inflammation of the vestibular organ and is most probably secondary to a virus. It is the inflammation that results in the sudden onset of severe vertigo with nausea and vomiting. Hearing loss and tinnitus may also be present. ➢ Treatment is symptomatic with a short course of vestibular sedative and gentle mobilisation. Patients should be told that further mild attacks may occur for a few months afterwards and therefore he or she should avoid situations where loss of balance could be dangerous. Recovery may be enhanced by graduated vestibular rehabilitation exercises. Some patients develop BPPV after acute labyrinthitis.
83	G	Demyelinating condition such as multiple sclerosis ➢ Internuclear ophthalmoplegia (INO) is a disorder of conjugate lateral gaze in which the affected eye shows impairment of adduction. When an attempt is made to gaze contralaterally (relative to the affected eye), the affected eye adducts minimally, if at all. The contralateral eye abducts, however with nystagmus Additionally, the divergence of the eyes leads to horizontal diplopia.

		➢ Internuclear ophthalmoplegia is classic for demyelinating condition such as multiple sclerosis. The symptoms of MS may mimic trigeminal neuralgia (TN) which is a neuropathic disorder characterized by episodes of intense pain in the face, originating from the trigeminal nerve. It is characterized by episodes of intense facial pain that last from a few sec to several minutes or hours. The episodes of intense pain may occur paroxysmally. Individual attacks usually affect one side of the face at a time, lasting from several seconds to a few minutes and repeat up to hundreds of times throughout the day. The pain also tends to occur in cycles with remissions lasting months or even years. 10–12% of cases are bilateral. Pain attacks are known to worsen in frequency or severity over time, in some patients. Some patients also experience pain in the index finger.
84	F	Common migraine ➢ Migraine is a chronic neurological disorder characterized by moderate to severe headaches and nausea. It is about three times more common in women than men.

		➢ Typical or classical migraine headache is unilateral (affecting one half of the head) and pulsating in nature and lasting from two to 72 hours; symptoms include nausea, vomiting and photophobia and are generally aggravated by routine activity. Approximately one-third of people who suffer from migraine headaches perceive an aura—transient visual, sensory, language, or motor disturbances signaling the migraine will soon occur. ➢ Common migraine is associated with phonophobia which is an increased sensitivity to sound. ➢ Migraine may sometimes mimic atypical Facial Pain (AFP), is regarded as a pathological entity involving a wide group of facial pain without a specific cause or known mechanism. Generally, this pain is neuropathic in presentation, consisting of burning, superficial or deep-aching, stabbing pain. AFP may also be described as poorly localized, typically involving the nose, eye, cheek, temple, and jaw.

		Additional notes ***Temporal arteritis*** - Temporal arteritis or Horton disease is an inflammatory disease of blood vessels most commonly involving large and medium arteries of the head. It is a form of vasculitis. - It is more common in Females than males by a ratio of 2:1 and more common in whites than black. The mean age of onset is > 55 years, and it is rare in those less than 55 years of age. - Patients present with: bruits; fever; headache; tenderness and sensitivity on the scalp; jaw claudication; tongue claudication ;reduced visual acuity; acute visual loss; diplopia; acute tinnitus ***Temporomandibular Joint dysfunction*** • TMJ dysfunction is an umbrella term covering acute or chronic inflammation of the temporomandibular joint, which connects the mandible to the skull. • The temporomandibular joint

			is susceptible to many of the conditions that affect other joints in the body, including ankylosis, arthritis, trauma, dislocations, developmental anomalies, neoplasia and reactive lesions. • Symptoms associated with TMJ disorders may be: Biting or chewing difficulty or discomfort; clicking, popping, or grating sound when opening or closing the mouth; Dull, aching pain in the face; Earache (particularly in the morning); Headache (particularly in the morning); Hearing loss; Migraine (particularly in the morning); Jaw pain or tenderness of the jaw; reduced ability to open or close the mouth. Tinnitus; Neck and shoulder pain; Dizziness. ***Cluster headaches*** • Occur periodically: spontaneous remissions interrupt active periods of pain. The cause of the disease is unknown. It affects 0.1% of

			the population, and men are more commonly affected. • Cluster headaches are excruciating unilateral headaches of extreme intensity. The duration of the common attack ranges from as short as 15 minutes to three hours or more. The onset of an attack is rapid, and most often without the preliminary signs that are characteristic of a migraine. However, some sufferers report preliminary sensations of pain in the general area of attack, often referred to as 'shadows', which may warn them an attack is lurking or imminent. • Though the headaches are almost exclusively unilateral, there are some documented as cases of 'side-shifting' between cluster periods, or, even rarer, simultaneously (within the same cluster period) bilateral headache. Trigeminal neuralgia headaches have similar qualities but the pain is mostly located around the facial area

		and is described as being like stabbing electric shocks, burning, pressing, crushing, exploding or shooting pain that becomes intractable. ***The sphenopalatine neuralgia*** • Characterized for a throbbing pain mostly unilateral encircling the orbit and occasionally extended to the neighboring areas, it is associated with rhinorrhoea, sneezing crisis and abnormal lacrimation.
85	I	Rochalimaea (or Bartonella) henselae ➢ *Bartonella henselae* is a proteobacterium that can cause bacteremia, endocarditis, bacillary angiomatosis, and peliosis hepatis. It is also the causative agent of cat-scratch disease (bartonellosis) which, as the name suggests occurs after a cat bite or scratch. ➢ The disease is characterized by lymphadenopathy (swelling of the lymph nodes) and fever. Peliosis hepatis caused by *B. henselae* can occur alone or develop with cutaneous bacillary angiomatosis or bacteremia. Patients with peliosis hepatitis present

with gastrointestinal symptoms, fever, chills, and an enlarged liver and spleen containing blood-filled cavities. This systemic disease can be seen in patients infected with HIV, or serve as a co-infection of those who have contracted Lyme disease, etc., and other immunocompromised individuals.

- *Bartonella henselae* is a member of the class of the *Bartonella* genus, one of the most common types of bacteria in the world. The presence of bacteria can be detected by a special stain called Warthin–Starry stain.
- *Bartonella* henselae (cat scratch disease) infections are usually sel*f*-limiting, but can be treated with azithromycin (macrolide) or doxycycline. This is the causative organism of cat scratch fever (bartonellosis). Symptoms include tender and swollen regional lymph nodes with occasional papules at the site of the bite. This may be associated with low grade fever and headache.
- Biopsy confirms follicular hyperplasia, suppurative granulomas with central stellate necrosis.

86	K	Streptococci milleri ➢ These are spherical Gram-positive bacteria which grow in chains and which are catalase negative. They are divided into alpha-haemolytic and beta-haemolytic, the latter of which are further divided into Lancefield groups (of which A and B are the most common and clinically important, hence group A beta-haemolytic Streptococci). ➢ A subset of Streptococcus viridans, but the species in this group differ in their haemolytic pattern and diseases caused. These species are often beta-haemolytic and produce pyogenic infections. ➢ Streptococcus milleri is a term used to refer to the Streptococcus intermedius group, which contains three distinct streptococcal species including Streptococcus intermedius, Streptococcus constellatus, and Streptococcus anginosus. These bacteria are found in the human oral cavity and have been associated with a variety of infections including bacteraemia; endocarditis; and CNS, oral, and thoracic infections.

87	F	Klebsiella rhinoscleromatis ➢ Klebsiella pneumoniae is a Gram-negative, non-motile, encapsulated, lactose fermenting, facultative anaerobic, rod shaped bacterium found in the normal flora of the mouth, skin, and intestines. It is clinically the most important member of the Klebsiella genus of Enterobacteriaceae. Seven species of the Klebsiella genus, with demonstrated similarities in DNA homology are known. These are (1) Klebsiella pneumoniae, (2) Klebsiella ozaenae, (3) Klebsiella terrigena, (4) Klebsiella rhinoscleromatis, (5) Klebsiella oxytoca, (6) Klebsiella planticola, and (7) Klebsiella ornithinolytica. ➢ Of these, K. oxytoca and K. rhinoscleromatis have also been demonstrated in human clinical specimens. In recent years, Klebsiella have become important pathogens in nosocomial infections. ➢ These organisms cause rhinoscleroma, a chronic granulomatous disease of the nose and occasionally lower respiratory tract that is most common in Central America and Eastern Europe. ➢ It has three key stages – catarrhal

			(characterized by rhinitis followed by mucopurulent rhinorrhoea), granulomatous (bluish red nasal mucosa and intranasal nodules causing epistaxis) and sclerotic (where granulomas coalesce in the nose, larynx and tracheobronchial tree). ➢ Diagnosis is by identification of nonspecific chronic inflammatory cells (Russell bodies) and vacuolated histiocytes (Mikulicz cells) on biopsy. ➢ K. pneumoniae can cause the disease Klebsiella pneumonia. They cause destructive changes to human lungs inflammation and hemorrhage with cell death (necrosis) that sometimes produces a thick, bloody, mucoid sputum (currant jelly sputum). Typically these bacteria gain access after a person aspirates colonising oropharyngeal microbes into the lower respiratory tract. As a general rule, Klebsiella infections are mostly seen in people with a weakened immune system. ➢ Two unusual infections of note are from Klebsiella are rhinoscleroma and ozena. Rhinoscleroma is a chronic inflammatory process involving the nasopharynx. Ozena is a chronic

		atrophic rhinitis that produces necrosis of nasal mucosa and mucopurulent nasal discharge. ➢ Treatment is with streptomycin or tetracycline.
88	D	Borrelia Burgdorferi ➢ This Gram-negative spirochete bacterium is the causative agent of Lyme disease, which is transmitted by ticks. Lyme disease is a zoonotic, vector-borne disease transmitted by ticks; the causative agent is named after the researcher Willy Burgdorfer, who first isolated the bacterium in 1982. ➢ *B. burgdorferi* is one of the few pathogenic bacteria that can survive without iron, having replaced all of its iron-sulfur cluster enzymes with enzymes that use manganese, thus avoiding the problem many pathogenic bacteria face in acquiring iron. ➢ It takes more than 24 hours of attachment for transfer of *B. burgdorferi*, making regular 'tick checks' helpful in preventing infection. ➢ *B. burgdorferi* infections have been linked to non-Hodgkin lymphomas. ➢ Lyme disease clinical features include the characteristic bull's eye rash and

		erythema chronicum migrans (a rash which spreads peripherally and spares the central part), as well as myocarditis, cardiomyopathy, arrhythmias, arthritis, arthralgia, meningitis, neuropathies and facial nerve palsy. Its clinical features include erythema chronicum migrans (usually at the site of initial infection), arthritis, meningitis, cranial neuropathies and facial nerve palsy.
89	H	Rhinosporidium Seeberi ➢ The organism causing rhinosporidioses was initially thought to be a fungus, but recently been re-classified as a parasite. ➢ Rhinosporidiosis is a chronic granulomatous disease that affects the nose and nasopharynx in 70% of cases and conjunctiva in 15%. This organism infects the mucosa of the nasal cavity resulting in lesion. ➢ The mass lesion appears to be polypoidal in nature with a granular surface speckled with whitish spores. The rhinosporidial lesion is similar to a strawberry or mulberry and may extend from the nasal cavity into the nasopharynx and oropharynx. ➢ These lesions commonly cause

		bleeding from the nasal cavity. The sites affected are nose (78%), nasopharynx (68%), tonsil (3%), eye (1%) and skin. *Rhinosporidium seeberi* can also affect the lacrimal gland and also rarely the skin of genitalia. ➢ Symptoms include nasal block, epistaxis and rhinorrhoea. Signs include strawberry nasal polyps and a granular mucosa. ➢ Diagnosis is on biopsy and treatment involves excision of large lesions or dapsone.
90	A	Olfactory nerve ➢ The olfactory nerve is the shortest of the twelve cranial nerves and only one of two cranial nerves (the other being the optic nerve) that do not join with the brainstem. ➢ The olfactory nerve filaments are bipolar and pass through the cribriform plate to synapse with the neurons in the olfactory bulb. These neurons in turn synapse with the olfactory cortex via the olfactory tract. Olfactory receptor neurons continue to be born throughout life and extend new axons to the olfactory bulb. Olfactory ensheathing glia wraps bundles of these axons and is thought to facilitate

		their passage into the central nervous system. ➢ The sense of smell (olfaction) arises from the stimulation of olfactory (or odorant) receptors by small molecules of different spatial, chemical, and electrical properties that pass over the nasal epithelium in the nasal cavity during inhalation. These interactions are transduced into electrical activity in the olfactory bulb, which then transmits the electrical activity to other parts of the olfactory system and the rest of the central nervous system via the olfactory tract.
91	D	Trochlear nerve ➢ The trochlear nerve (the fourth cranial nerve, also called the fourth nerve, IV) is a motor nerve (a 'somatic efferent' nerve) that innervates a single muscle: the superior oblique muscle of the eye. ➢ The trochlear nerve is unique among the cranial nerves in several respects. It is the smallest nerve in terms of the number of axons it contains. It has the greatest intracranial length. Other than the optic nerve (cranial nerve II), it is the only cranial nerve that decussates (crosses to the other side) before innervating its target. It is the only

		cranial nerve that exits from the dorsal aspect of the brainstem.
92	I	Glossopharyngeal nerve ➢ The glossopharyngeal nerve has only one somatic motor function and that is innervation of the stylopharyngeus. However, it also supplies taste on the posterior third of the tongue and chemical perception at the carotid bodies. ➢ The glossopharyngeal nerve is the ninth (IX) of twelve pairs of cranial nerves (24 nerves total). It exits the brainstem out from the sides of the upper medulla, just rostral (closer to the nose) to the vagus nerve. ➢ The motor division of the glossopharyngeal nerve is derived from the basal plate of the embryonic medulla oblongata, while the sensory division originates from the cranial neural crest. ➢ There are a number of functions of the glossopharyngeal nerve; It receives general sensory fibers (ventral trigeminothalamic tract) from the tonsils, the pharynx, the middle ear and the posterior 1/3 of the tongue; It receives special sensory fibers (taste) from the posterior one-third of the

		tongue; It receives visceral sensory fibers from the carotid bodies, carotid sinus; It supplies parasympathetic fibers to the parotid gland via the otic ganglion.
93	I	Glossopharyngeal nerve ➢ The glossopharyngeal nerve also has a secretomotor function, and it exerts this on the parotid gland. The tympanic portion leaves the glossopharyngeal nerve when still in the jugular foramen. The tympanic branch then passes through the inferior tympanic canaliculus into the tympanic cavity where it forms the tympanic plexus. It reenters the skull to become the lesser petrosal nerve. This nerve travels alongside the greater petrosal nerve until its exit at the foramen ovale. It joins the otic ganglion and then via the auriculotemporal nerve innervates the parotid gland.
94	E	Trigeminal nerve ➢ The trigeminal nerve contains both sensory and motor fibres. It is responsible for sensation in the face and certain motor functions such as biting, chewing, and swallowing. ➢ The motor division of the trigeminal nerve is derived from the basal plate of

the embryonic pons, while the sensory division originates from the cranial neural crest.

- Somatic motor functions include supply to anterior belly of digastric, mylohyoid, tensor veli palatini, tensor tympani and the muscles of mastication.
- Unlike dermatomes in the rest of the body which show considerable overlap, the areas of cutaneous distribution of the three branches of the trigeminal nerve have sharp borders with relatively little overlap. Hence injection of local anesthetics results in the complete loss of sensation from well–defined areas of the face and mouth. For example, the teeth on one side of the jaw can be numbed by injecting the mandibular nerve.
- The ophthalmic, maxillary and mandibular branches of the trigeminal nerve leave the skull through three separate foramina: the superior orbital fissure, the foramen rotundum and the foramen ovale. The mnemonic *__S__tanding __R__oom __O__nly* can be used to remember that V1 passes through the superior orbital fissure, V2 through the foramen rotundum, and V3 through

		the foramen ovale. ➢ The *ophthalmic nerve* (V1) carries sensory information from the scalp and forehead, the upper eyelid, the conjunctiva and cornea of the eye, the nose (including the tip of the nose, except alae nasi), the nasal mucosa, the frontal sinuses, and parts of the meninges (the dura and blood vessels). ➢ The *maxillary nerve* (V2) carries sensory information from the lower eyelid and cheek, the nares and upper lip, the upper teeth and gums, the nasal mucosa, the palate and roof of the pharynx, the maxillary, ethmoid and sphenoid sinuses, and parts of the meninges. ➢ The *mandibular nerve* (V3) carries sensory information from the lower lip, the lower teeth and gums, the chin and jaw (except the angle of the jaw, which is supplied by C2–C3), parts of the external ear, and parts of the meninges. The mandibular nerve carries touch/position and pain/temperature sensation from the mouth.
95	B	Left Ménière's disease. ➢ Ménière's is a clinical diagnosis. However, it can be aided by

electrocochleography which shows a large summating potential in relation to the action potential. This is thought to occur secondary to hydrops. A ratio of greater than 0.5 is used to aid diagnosis.

- Electrocochleography (ECochG) is a technique of recording stimulus-related responses or electrical potentials of the inner ear and auditory nerve. Components potentials of the human electrocochleogram are: cochlear microphonics (CM), summating potentials (SM), and action potential (AP). These potentials can either be recorded independently or in various combinations.
- CM and SP are generated in the organ of Corti and are a type of receptor potential. AP is the neural potentials generated by the cochlear nerve.
- Electrodes can be either invasive of non-invasive. Invasive electrodes like transtympanic needle give clearer, more robust electrical response (larger amplitudes) since the electrodes are very close to the generators. The needle is placed on the promontory wall of the middle ear and the round window. Non-invasive electrodes or

		the extratympanic electrodes can be used atraumatically without causing pain or discomfort to the patient. Unlike the invasive electrodes, there is no need for sedation, anesthetics and medical supervision to use non-invasive electrodes. The responses, however, are smaller in magnitude. Some of the commercially available ear canal electrodes are foam earplug, eartrode and tiptrode.
96	A	Left labyrinthitis obliterans ➢ Labyrinthitis obliterans can occur from chronic otitis media, cochlear otosclerosis, meningitis or measles. ➢ The CT shows calcification of the membranous labyrinth. Because of labyrinthitis obliterans, it is important to implant patients early with cochlear implant following meningitis. ➢ However, there is a significant negative correlation between spiral ganglion cell survival and the presence of bony occlusion of the inner ear. This raises the question as to whether patients with extensive ossification are likely to show significant benefit from cochlear implant. CT scanning is not totally reliable for diagnosing labyrinthitis obliterans and occasionally the

		condition may be mistaken for a Michel anomaly. T2 weighted MRI may also be needed.
97	C	Left otosclerosis ➢ Otosclerosis is a progressive genetic condition of the otic capsule characterised by abnormal bone remodelling. This leads primarily to fixation of the stapes footplate, although other sites such as the round window niche and cochlear wall may be involved. ➢ Involvement of the oval window typically results in a conductive hearing loss whilst cochlear otosclerosis leads to sensorineural hearing loss. ➢ High resolution CT scanning may show the extent of otospongiosis just anterior to the oval window. Involvement of the cochlear gives rise to the 'double density sign' on CT. ➢ Therapeutic options include hearing aid or sodium fluoride and surgical intervention (stapedectomy or stapedotomy). ➢ A speech audiogram, to check the cochlear reserve, is important before considering surgery. ➢ Cochlear implant may be considered in patient with severe SNHL secondary to

		cochlear otosclerosis. Recent developments in semi-implantable and fully implantable middle ear implants provide an alternative where air conduction aids are not tolerated or where previous ossiculoplasty surgery has been inadequate.
98	A	Chi square test ➢ This is an example of count data. The χ^2 test is used to determine whether there is a difference between expected frequencies in one or more categories. One would need to count the number of successful and unsuccessful candidates from Boston. ➢ The χ^2 distribution (also χ^2 or χ^2-distribution) with *k* degrees of freedom is the distribution of a sum of the squares of *k* independent standard normal random variables. ➢ It is one of the most widely used probability distributions in inferential statistics, e.g. in hypothesis testing or in construction of confidence intervals. When there is a need to contrast it with the noncentral χ^2 distribution, this distribution is sometimes called the central χ^2distribution. ➢ The χ^2distribution is used in the common χ^2tests for goodness of fit of

		an observed distribution to a theoretical one, the independence of two criteria of classification of qualitative data, and in confidence interval estimation for a population standard deviation of a normal distribution from a sample standard deviation. ➢ Many other statistical tests also use this distribution, like Friedman's analysis of variance by ranks. The χ^2distribution is a special case of the gamma distribution.
99	J	Pearson's correlation coefficient ➢ Pearson's correlation coefficient is a technique for investigating the relationship between two quantitative, continuous variables, for example, age and blood pressure. ➢ Pearson's correlation coefficient (r) is a measure of the strength of the association between the two variables. Here you are asked to assess a possible association between two different variables, so you need either Pearson's or Spearman's correlation coefficient. Blood pressure and age are normally distributed, hence Pearson.
100	K	Spearman's correlation coefficient ➢ Here again you are asked to assess a

			possible association between two different variables (air conduction thresholds and age). Therefore you need a correlation test. The former is not normally distributed so Spearman's is a non-parametric measure of statistical dependance between two variables. ➢ The Spearman's correlation coefficient is often described as being 'nonparametric.' This can have two meanings. First, the fact that a perfect Spearman correlation results when X and Y are related by any monotonic function can be contrasted with the Pearson correlation, which only gives a perfect value when X and Y are related by a linear function. The other sense in which the Spearman correlation is non-parametric in that its exact sampling distribution can be obtained without requiring knowledge (i.e., knowing the parameters) of the joint probability distribution of X and Y. It assesses how well the relationship between two variables can be described using a monotonic function.

CHAPTER 3

Paper 3

EMI Questions (Q1-Q100)

For each stem, select one correct answer option.

Theme: Watering eye

Options for Questions 1–2:

A Blepharitis
B Canalicular stenosis
C Conjunctival disease
D Ectropion
E Nasolacrimal duct blockage
F Punctal stenosis

For each of the following cases, select the single most likely diagnosis. Each option may be used once, more than once or not at all.

1. A 78-year-old female presents with epiphora following excision of a basal cell carcinoma from beneath her left eye. Examination shows tension and eversion of the lower eyelid.

2. A 78-year-old woman presents with a watery eye. Lacrimal syringing of the lower punctum shows reflux from the upper punctum but no penetration into the nose.

Theme: Nerve injury/dysfunction

Options for Questions 3–5:

A Short sphenopalatine nerve
B Anterior palatine nerve
C Anterior superior alveolar nerve
D Long sphenopalatine nerve
E Middle palatine nerve
F Lingual nerve
G Greater auricular nerve
H Facial nerve
I Ophthalmic nerve
J Spinal accessory nerve
K Chorda tympani
L Hypoglossal nerve
M Glossopharyngeal nerve
N Cervical sympathetic plexus

For each of the clinical vignette listed below, select the most likely nerve to be involved from the above list. Each of the listed options may be used once, more than once or not at all.

3. A 48-year-old male presents with numbness of the upper left medial incisor following transantral surgery on his pterygopalatine fossa.

4. A 35-year-old male presents complaining of loss of taste on the left side of his tongue and severe bleeding from the left side of his tongue which he has bitten. Three days previously he had a left lower impacted wisdom tooth extraction.

5. A 75-year-old woman presents complaining of clouding vision in her left eye after developing a rash over her left forehead. She also mentions a burning pain over her left forehead and her left eye. Examination reveals no ptosis or diplopia and the corneal reflex is intact.

Theme: Tinnitus

Options for Questions 6–10:

A Arterial malformation
B Carotid stenosis
C CT angiogram
D Dural arteriovenous fistula
E Glomus jugulare
F Glomus tympanicum
G MRI with gadolinium
H Palatal myoclonus
I Patulous Eustachian tube
J Spontaneous otoacoustic emissions
K Stapedius myoclonus
L Superior semicircular canal dehiscence
M Tensor tympani myoclonus
N Venous malformation

For each of the following cases, select the single most likely diagnosis. Each option may be used once, more than once or not at all.

6. A 32-year-old female presents with thumping tinnitus. It is exacerbated by external noise. Examination shows objective tinnitus that the

examiner can appreciate. Review of the tympanic membrane shows movement in synchrony to the tinnitus.

7. A 52-year-old female presents with unilateral pulsatile tinnitus, and conductive hearing loss. CT scan with contrast shows a vascular mass filling the epitypanum and mastoid cavity

8. A 65-year-old male presents with recent weight loss describes a blowing tinnitus and echo sensation of his own voice. He admits his symptoms resolve when he has a cold and nasal blockage. Tympanometry shows frequent fluctuations in the trace.

9. A 45-year-old man presents complaining of hearing loss. Examination reveals an audible noise tinnitus which the patient was unaware of.

10. A 45-year-old man presents complaining of pulsatile noise in his left ear. The noise decreases when he performs a Valsalva manoeuvre.

Theme: TNM classification

Options for Questions 11–13:

A T1N0M0
B T2N0M0
C T3N0M0
D T4N0M0
E T1N1M0
F T2N1M0
G T1N2M1

H T2N2M1
I T3N2M1
J T4N2M1

For each of the following cases, select the single most appropriate TNM stage. Each option may be used once, more than once or not at all.

11. A 64-year-old man presents with a tumour of the larynx, which extends into the subglottis. Examination reveals a single unilateral node that is about 1.5 cm in size. No metastases are evident on CT/MRI.

12. A 54-year-old woman presents with a tumour confined to a mobile left vocal cord, but no palpable cervical nodes.

13. A 78-year-old man presents with an advanced tumour extending beyond the larynx into the trachea. Examination reveals multiple nodes on the left the largest measures 5cm. He also has enlarged nodes on his chest CT.

Theme: Nasal blockage

Options for Questions 14–17:

A Atrophic rhinitis
B Deviation of nasal bones
C Deviation of nasal septum
D Encephalocoele
E Foreign body
F Mucocoele

G Nasal polyps
H Nasolabial cyst
I Nasopharyngeal carcinoma
J Perennial allergic rhinitis
K Removal of inferior turbinates
L Rhinitis medicamentosa
M Rhinolith
N Wegener's granulomatosis

For each of the following cases, select the single most likely diagnosis. Each option may be used once, more than once or not at all.

14. A 64-year-old man presents with a history of bilateral nasal blockage. He has derived temporary relief with an 'over-the-counter' decongestant from the pharmacy, which he has been using consistently for 3 months.

15. A 20-year-old man presents complaining of a persistent right-sided nasal obstruction. He underwent a manipulation under anaesthetic 10 days after nasal trauma.

16. A 25-year-old man presents with gradual blockage of both nostrils. The GP examined the nose and noted pale insensate swelling in bilaterally. The patient is also asthmatic and sensitive to aspirin.

17. A 3-year-old boy presents with an offensive unilateral nasal discharge.

Theme: Advice

Options for Questions 18–22:

A Avoid contact sports
B Change contraceptive pill
C Continue as before
D Do not immerse in water
E Doctor to inform DVLA
F Gargle saline
G Lose weight
H Note and adhere to the sell by dates on food
I Patient to inform DVLA
J Pinch the alar region of the nose and lean forward
K Place icepacks on forehead
L Reduced salt in diet
M Stop drinking
N Stop smoking

For each of the following cases, select the single most appropriate advice. Each option may be used once, more than once or not at all.

18. A 17-year-old male rugby player presents with a positive monospot-test, and a palpable mass below the costal margin on the left hand side of the abdomen.

19. A 49-year-old female lorry driver presents with snoring. A sleep study shows an apnoea-hypopnea index of greater than 30.

20. A 78-year-old woman presents with anosmia and ageusia following a severe cold. MR and CT scanning are reported as normal.

21. A 35-year-old man who has had subcutaneous Vicryl sutures used to close his wound after a total thyroidectomy.

22. A 36-year-old overweight woman presents with episodic vertigo, hearing loss, tinnitus and fullness in her right ear.

Theme: Nerve damage during neck operation

Options for Questions 23–27:

A C1
B C2
C C3
D C4
E C5
F C6
G C7
H C8
I C5–C7 (Long thoracic nerve of Bell)
J T1
K T2
L T1–L2 (sympathetic chain)
M Vagus nerve

For each of the following cases, select the single most likely nerve. Each option may be used once, more than once or not at all.

23. A 39-year-old woman presents four weeks following an operation on the neck, unable to flex the metacarpophalangeal joints. There also appears to be wasting of the dorsal interossei muscles.

24. A 39-year-old woman presents with ipsilateral drooping of the eyelid and dilated pupils, 2 days after a neck dissection.

25. A 39-year-old woman presents with numbness over the lateral surface of his upper arm, 10 days after a neck dissection.

26. A 39-year-old woman presents complaining of paraesthesia on the medial aspect of the forearm, 2 weeks after neck dissection.

27. A 39-year-old woman presents complains of her scapula protruding when she pushes open a door, 4 weeks after a neck dissection.

Theme: Antibiotic usage

Options for Questions 28–34

A IV benzylpenicillin
B IV cefotaxime
C IV co-amoxiclav
D IV metronidazole
E Oral amoxicillin
F Oral clarithromycin
G Oral co-amoxiclav
H Oral erythromycin
I Oral metronidazole

J Oral penicillin V

For each of the following cases, select the single most appropriate diagnosis. Each option may be used once, more than once or not at all.

28. A 5-year-old boy presents to his GP with inflamed tonsils and pyrexia of 37.5 C. He is able to eat and drink. Blood test reveals a neutrophilia.

29. A 17-year-old girl presents with lymphadenopathy and a rash after receiving a prescription from her GP for a sore throat.

30. A 17-year-old girl presents with quinsy and difficulty swallowing. The ENT registrar recommended anaerobic cover in addition to benzylpenicillin.

31. A 4-year-old boy presents with epiglottitis.

Theme: Arterial blood gases

	A	B	C	D	E	F
pH	7.36	7.5	7.4	7	7.5	7
PaO2 (kPa)	7.9	13.8	11	5.1	12.1	12.4
PaCO2 (kPa)	4.2	2.7	5.2	7.8	3.2	2.1
$HCO3^-$	22	23	25	19	23	14

Normal values:pH:7.35–7.45; Partial Pressure of Oxygen:(Pa02) >11 kPa; Partial Pressure of Carbon Dioxide:(PaC02) 4.7–6.0 kPa;

Bicarbonate:(HCO3-) 21–28 mmol/L.

For each of the following cases, select the single most appropriate arterial blood gas result. Each option may be used once, more than once or not at all.

32. A 16-year-old girl presents to accident and emergency by ambulance from a music festival. She complains of acute onset of shortness of breath and atypical chest pain. On examination her respiratory rate is 30, she anxious and has carpopedal spasm.

33. A 25-year-old man presents with a reduced GCS of 9 to accident and emergency. He is a known insulin dependent diabetic. He has been unwell and not eating for the last few days. He is breathing deeply and his breath smells of pears.

34. A 72-year-old male presents collapsed on the ward. An ECG shows ventricular fibrillation. He deteriorates and becomes asystolic after four cycles of resuscitation. An arterial blood gas sample is taken during resuscitation while the patient is being ventilated using a bag and mask.

Theme: Calculation of local anaesthetic

Options for Questions 35–38:

A 2 mL
B 3 mL
C 4 mL
D 6 mL
E 8 mL
F 10 mL

G 20 mL
H 40 mL
I 80 mL
J 100 mL
K 200 mL
L 300 mL
M 400 mL
N 500 mL

Select the volume of saline needed from the above list to make the following solution. Each option may be used once, more than once or not at all.

35 To make 1:200,000 solution using 1 mL of 1:1000 adrenaline.

36. To make the safe maximum dose of 1% lignocaine for a 70 kg man.

37. To make a solution containing 200 mg of 5% cocaine.

38. To make 1:80,000 solution containing 0.125 mg of adrenaline.

Theme: Oral lesions

Options for Questions 39–41:

A Actinomycosis
B Amyloidosis
C Aphthous Ulcer
D Behçet's disease
E Bullous Pemphigoid
F Hairy Leukoplakia

G Lichen planus
H Oral candidiasis
I Squamous Papilloma
J Syphilitic ulcer
K Torus palatinus
L Traumatic ulcer

For each of the following cases, select the single most likely diagnosis. Each option may be used once, more than once or not at all.

39. A 25-year-old man presents with a single painful white lesion on his gingiva, measuring about 2 mm in diameter.

40. An 18-year-old girl presents with a well demarcated benign lesion on her uvula.

41. A 29-year-old man presents with a lesion associated with an anaerobic gram-negative bacterium that produces sulphur like granules.

Theme: Eponyms

Options for Questions 42–46:

A Alexander's law
B Arnold nerve
C Arnold's reflex
D Boyce sign
E Bryce sign
F Grisel sign
G Hennebert
H Melkersson–Rosenthal syndrome

I Trotter's method
J Trotter's syndrome
K Tullio's phenomena
L Woodruff's plexus

For each of the following cases, select the single most likely diagnosis. Each option may be used once, more than once or not at all.

42. A 76-year-old man presents with deafness and neuralgia affecting his face on the right side. He is experiencing nasal regurgitation and difficulty in speaking. He has a mass on CT in the nasopharynx.

43. A 45-year-old woman presents with nystagmus, which increases in intensity when she looks to the left and decreases on gaze to the right. She has a vestibular lesion on the left.

44. A 34-year-old male diver presents with nausea and vertigo on hearing a loud noise.

45. A 5-year-old boy presents with torticollis, with a flexed and rotated head following adenoidectomy.

46. A 65-year-old male patient presents with dysphagia and a mass in the neck that gurgles on palpation.

Theme: Infectious diseases

Options for Questions 47–51:

A Chickenpox
B Cytomegalovirus infection
C Erythema infectiosum (slapped cheek disease)

D Hand, foot and mouth disease
E Infectious mononucleosis
F Kawasaki
G Lyme
H Measles
I Mumps
J Rubella
K Scarlet fever
L Steven–Johnson syndrome
M Tonsillitis
N Toxoplasmosis

For each set of the following cases, select the single most likely infectious disease. Each option may be used once, more than once or not at all.

47. A 10-year-old girl presents with red spots on the buccal mucosa, conjunctivitis, otitis media, rhinitis and maculopapular rash

48. A 10-year-old girl presents with fever, conjunctivitis, fissuring of the lips, strawberry tongue, swelling of the extremities, cervical lymphadenopathy and peripheral desquamation of the palms and soles of the feet

49 A 14-year-old male presents with fever, sore throat, coated tonsils, malaise, wide spread lymphadenopathy and tender abdomen

50. A 12-year-old female presents with sudden onset of sore throat headache, fever and a scarlet blush rash that fades with direct pressure. Desquamation occurs

after a few days, especially on the feet and hands. Tonsillar inflammation is also present.

51. A 21-year-old man presents with sudden onset of conjunctival, nasal, genital lesions, and exfoliating lesions on the hand and feet, following sulphonamide therapy.

Theme: Tuning fork testing

Options for Questions 52–53:

A Bilateral conductive hearing loss
B Bilateral sensorineural hearing loss
C Conductive hearing loss left side
D Conductive hearing loss right side
E Normal hearing
F Sensorineural hearing loss left side
G Sensorineural hearing loss right side

For each of the following tuning fork test results, select the single most appropriate interpretation. Each option may be used once, more than once or not at all.

52. In a tuning fork test, Weber's does not localise to either side, whilst Rinne's is positive bilaterally.

53. In a tuning fork test, Weber's localises to the left, whilst Rinne's is positive on both sides.

Theme: Bony landmarks on the skull

Options for Questions 54–57:

A Asterion

B Bregma
C Inion
D Lambda
E Nasion
F Pterion
G Rhinion
H Spine of Henlé

For each of the following skull descriptions, select the single most likely bony landmark. Each option may be used once, more than once or not at all.

54. The point on the skull corresponding to the posterior end of the parietomastoid suture.

55. The landmark for the anterior branch of the middle meningeal artery, which underlies this area inside the skull

56. An important landmark for mastoid surgery.

57. The highest point of the external occipital protuberance.

Theme: Medical conditions relevant to otolaryngology

Options for Questions 58–60:

A Ankylosing spondylitis
B Carcinoma of the bronchus
C Churg–Strauss syndrome
D Ehlers–Danlos syndrome
E Hyperthyroidism

F Parathyroid hyperplasia
G Pneumonia
H Relapsing polychondritis
I Rheumatoid arthritis
J Sarcoidosis
K Syphilis
L Tuberculosis
M Wegener's

For each of the following cases, select the single most likely diagnosis. Each option may be used once, more than once or not at all.

58. A 50-year-old male patient presents with chronic sinusitis. Recently he complained of bloody nasal discharge, cough and shortness of breath. The chest X ray shows a diffuse area of consolidation and cavities in the right middle and left upper lobe. Urinalysis shows red blood cells cast and protein

59. A 50-year-old female patient present with a two-year history of a hoarse voice, and some difficulty breathing, which she felt, was normal for her age. Examination reveals a bluish colouration on her nose, and flexible nasendoscopy shows a smooth benign looking supraglottic lesion. Blood tests reveal calcium of 3.8 mmol/L

60. A 52-year-old man presents with a septal perforation. He makes regular overseas business trips.

Theme: Haematological and biochemical investigations

Options for Questions 61–65:

A ACE
B Blood glucose
C Bone profile
D c-ANCA
E Fasting lipids
F Full blood count
G Liver function test
H MPO
I p-ANCA
J PR3
K RAST
L Serum and urine osmolality
M Thyroid function test
N Urea and electrolytes

For each of the following cases, select the single most appropriate investigation. Each option may be used once, more than once or not at all.

61. A75-year-old man present with hearing loss. He is currently receiving cisplatin for a T3N0 laryngeal carcinoma.

62. A 35-year-old woman presents with bruising. She is taking sodium valproate for vertebrobasilar migraine.

63. A 45-year-old man presents following a road traffic accident. Within 48 hours of the accident, he

complains of severe headache and passing excessive amounts of urine.

64. A 23-year-old woman presents with dermatographism complains of excessive sneezing and runny nose.

65. A 37-year-old woman presents with pyrexia of unknown origin in association with a diffuse painless right sided parotid swelling, right facial nerve palsy, hilar lymphadenopathy and nasal crusting with streaks of blood in nasal mucus

Theme: Microbiological pathogens

Options for Questions 66–70:

A Actinomyces israellii
B Bacteroides spp
C Bordetella pertussis
D Candida
E Coagulase negative staphylococci
F Haemophilus influenzae
G Klebsiellia
H Moxella catarrhalis
I MRSA
J Pseudomonas aeruginosa
K Staphylococcus aureus
L Streptococcus milleri
M Streptococcus pneumoniae

For each of the following cases, select the single most likely pathogen. Each option may be used once, more than once or not at all.

66. A 16-year-old boy presents with severe left-sided maxillary sinusitis following an upper respiratory tract infection.

67. A 15-year-old girl with cystic fibrosis develops a chest infection.

68. A 19-year-old woman presents with itchy ears. A microbiological swab is taken and the report came back stating a bacterium that commonly colonises human skin and mucosa.

69. A 39-year-old Egyptian woman presents with signs and symptoms consistent with atrophic rhinitis.

70. A 4-year-old Somalian boy presents in casualty with rapid onset of stridor and drooling. He has never been vaccinated.

Theme: Genetic disorders

Options for Questions 71–72:

A Cystic fibrosis
B Down's syndrome
C Haemophilia A
D Klinefelter's syndrome
E Neurofibromatosis type 1
F Osteogenesis imperfect
G Prader–Willi Syndrome

H Retinoblastoma
I Thalassemia trait
J Trisomy 13
K Trisomy 18
L Turner syndrome

For each of the following cases, select the single most likely genetic condition. Each option may be used once, more than once or not at all.

71. A 10-year-old Greek boy presents for genetic screening because of a suspected clotting disorder. The result reveals a common X-linked single gene disorder that affects clotting.

72. A 10-year-old Greek boy presents for genetic screening because of anaemia. The result reveals a common single gene disorder.

Theme: TNM staging

Options for Questions 73–75:

A T1N0
B T1N1
C T1N1a
D T1N1b
E T2N0
F T2N1M0
G T2N2aM0
H T2N2bM0
I T2N2cM0
J T2N3M0

K T3N0M0

L T3N1M0

M T4N0M0

N T4N1M0

For each of the following cases, select the single most appropriate TNM stage. Each option may be used once, more than once or not at all.

73. A 40-year-old barmaid presents with a 4-month history of a right throat discomfort. Examination reveals an indurated firm lesion in the right tonsil, measuring 1.5cm, and a 2.5 cm ipsilateral solitary lymph node in level 2 of the neck.

74. A 40-year-old barmaid presents with a 4-month history of a right throat discomfort. Examination reveals an indurated firm lesion in the right tonsil measuring 2.5cm, and a single ipsilateral lymph node, more than 3 cm, but not more than 6 cm in greatest dimension in level 2 of the neck.

75. A 40-year-old barmaid presents with a 4-month history of a right throat discomfort. Examination reveals an indurated firm lesion in the right tonsil measuring 3 cm, and a lymph node more than 6 cm in greatest dimension in level 2 of the neck.

Theme: Genetic terms

Options for Questions 76–80:

A Allele

B Genotype

C Meiosis
D Mitosis
E Mosaicism
F Non-disjunction
G Oncogene
H Phenotype
I Protooncogene
J Robertsonian translocation
K Translocation
L Trisomy
M Tumour suppressor gene
N Wild type

For each of the following genetic descriptions, select the single most appropriate genetic term. Each option may be used once, more than once or not at all.

76. The failure of two members of a chromosome pair to separate during meiosis.

77. A normal gene involved in the regulation of cell growth.

78. One of the alternative versions of a gene that can occupy a specific locus.

79. Cell division occurring in the germ cell.

80. The observed physical characteristics of an individual.

Theme: Hearing loss

Options for Questions 81–85:

A Benign intracranial hypertension

B Cochlear hydrops
C Cochlear otosclerosis
D Cogan's syndrome
E Enlarged vestibular aqueduct syndrome
F Heredito-degenerative disease of the cochlea
G Inner ear conductive presbyacusis
H Neural presbyacusis
I Sensory presbyacusis
J Strial presbyacusis
K Syphilitic ear
L Usher's syndrome

For each of the following cases, select the single most likely diagnosis. Each option may be used once, more than once or not at all.

81. A 52-year-old woman presents with a gradual hearing loss, showing a moderate slope towards the high frequencies but disproportionately severe decrease in speech discrimination.

82. A 56-year-old man presents with a bilateral symmetrical sensorineural loss showing a virtually flat line across all frequencies and well-preserved speech discrimination.

83. A 10-year-old boy presents with progressive sensorineural hearing loss, which suddenly worsens following head trauma whilst playing rugby.

84. A 66-year-old man presents with abrupt sensorineural hearing loss in the high frequencies and moderate speech discrimination.

85. A 70-year-old woman presents with bilateral symmetric sensorineural loss with an upward slope toward the high frequencies and preserved speech discrimination.

Theme: Tympanometry

Options for Questions 86–88:

A Type A
B Type Ad
C Type As
D Type B
E Type C1
F Type C2

For each of the following cases, select the single most likely tympanogram. Each option may be used once, more than once or not at all.

86. A 25-year-old man presents with suspicion of otitis media with effusion. Tympanometry reveals peak compliance less than -200 daPa.

87. A 25-year-old man presents with hearing loss after a falling from a ladder. Tympanometry reveals peak compliance is between -100 and +100 da Pa, but the reading was off the y-axis

88. A 25-year-old man presents with hearing loss. Audiometry was consistent with otosclerosis.

Theme: Biomaterials used in ENT

Options for Questions 89–93:

A	Ceramic
B	Copper
C	Gore-Tex
D	Gutta percha
E	Hydroxylapatite
F	Medpor
G	Plaster of Paris
H	Platinum
I	Silastic
J	Stainless steel
K	Surgisis
L	Teflon
M	Titanium

For each of the following cases, select the single most appropriate biomaterial. Each option may be used once, more than once or not at all.

89. A 16-year-old male with Treacher–Collins syndrome, and grade 3 microtia. The patient requires a prosthetic ear fixed on.

90. A 76-year-old man underwent unilateral resection of the upper jaw for carcinoma of the maxillary sinus. He requires a biomaterial to support the soft tissues of the cheek

91. A 40-year-old man presents with dizziness whilst swimming. Two years ago he had a modified radical mastoidectomy for cholesteatoma. The patient

requested obliteration of his mastoid cavity to avoid the caloric effect of water whilst swimming.

92. A 25-year-old woman presents with a unilateral conductive hearing loss following pregnancy. Clinical examination and investigation suggest a diagnosis of otosclerosis. The patient opted for surgery, and the surgeon chose to use a stapes prosthesis that has 'intrinsic memory'

93. A 12-year-old girl presents with bilateral profound sensorineural hearing following meningitis and now requires bilateral cochlear implants. The father is a biomaterial engineer and would like to know about the material used to make the cochlear implant electrode.

Theme: Paediatric hearing assessment

Options for Questions 94–97:

A Auditory brainstem response (ABR)
B Condition reflex audiometry
C Cortical evoked response audiometry
D Distraction test
E Otoacoustic emission
F Pure tone audiometry
G Speech discrimination test
H Tone decay test
I Tympanometry
J VEMP
K Visual reinforcement audiometry

For each of the following cases, select the single most appropriate investigation. Each option may be used once, more than once or not at all.

94. A 2-year-old girl presents with suspicion of a hearing loss.

95. A 5-month-old boy present with failed automated and manual OAE tests.

96. A 5-year-old boy presents with suspicion of a hearing loss.

97. A 4-month-old with suspicion of hearing loss.

Theme: Statistical testings

Options for Questions 98–100:

A Chi-squared (χ2) test
B Fisher's exact-test
C Friedman test
D F-test
E Kruskal–Wallis test
F Mann–Whitney U test
G McNemar
H One sample (paired) Student's t-test
I One-way analysis of variance (ANOVA)
J Pearsons correlation coefficient
K Spearman's rank correlation coefficient
L Two sample (unpaired) Student's t-test
M Two-way analysis of variance (ANOVA)
N Wilcoxon matched pairs test

For each of the following data sets, select the single most suitable statistical test. Each of the listed options may be used once, more than once or not at all.

98. To assess whether serum calcium changes twelve hours, one day and three days following total thyroidectomy, is affected by the rank of surgeons.

99. To compare the systolic BP measurements of four independent groups (n=80)/group of subjects.

100. Comparing DO-HNS exam scores between the north and south of England.

Answer Keys to Chapter 3 EMIs

<table>
<tr><td>1</td><td>D</td><td>Ectropion<ul><li>Epiphora can be caused by lid malposition. Ectropion or entropion (i.e. lid eversion or inversion respectively) will cause the puncta to malposition in the tear lake.</li><li>Ectropion can be congenital or acquired. If congenital the commonest cause is absence of the anterior lamella and is associated with Down's syndrome.</li><li>Acquired ectropion can be caused by advancing age causing involution, repetitive rubbing of eyes causing laxity, tethering skin cancers and facial nerve palsies. It can be classified into punctual, medial, lateral or tarsal (complete).</li><li>Treatment includes eye lubrication to prevent ulceration and surgical correction to help reposition the puncta, which is performed through a tightening procedure.</li></ul></td></tr>
<tr><td>2</td><td>E</td><td>Nasolacrimal duct blockage<ul><li>Watering eyes or epiphora is frequently referred to ENT by Ophthalmology for consideration of</li></ul></td></tr>
</table>

		endoscopic dacryocystorhinostomy to treat nasolacrimal duct blockage. ➢ Epiphora caused by nasolacrimal duct blockage responds best to endoscopic dacryocystorhinostomy. If syringing of fluid through the inferior punctum shows no passage of fluid into the nose but egress through the superior punctum it implies the inferior punctum, common canaliculus and superior punctum are all patent. If fluid cannot be syringed into the inferior punctum at all then there is a blockage in the inferior canaliculus. This will not be amenable to endoscopic dacryocystorhinostomy (DCR). ➢ Endoscopic DCR involves making an incision anterior to the middle turbinate and raising a mucosal flap. The groove between the uncinate and the lacrimal bone is found by advancing the flap posteriorly. Bone is removed in the groove using a bone punch and burr until there is wide exposure of the lacrimal sac. An incision into the sac is made. The puncta of the eyelids are cannulated with a needle threaded with a stent, to prevent stoma closure during healing. ➢ Success rates for endoscopic DCR are

		around 80-90%. If the treatment fails a repeat procedure can be planned or it can be done via an open approach. This has the advantage of assessing the proximal draining system, which may need surgical correction also.
3	C	Anterior superior alveolar nerve ➢ The anterior superior alveolar branch (anterior superior dental branch) arises from the maxillary nerve just before its exit from the infraorbital foramen; it descends in a canal in the anterior wall of the maxillary sinus, and divides into branches which supply the incisor and canine teeth. It communicates with the middle superior alveolar branch, and gives off a nasal branch, which passes through a minute canal in the lateral wall of the inferior meatus, and supplies the mucous membrane of the anterior part of the inferior meatus and the floor of the nasal cavity, communicating with the nasal. ➢ The anterior palatine nerve (greater palatine nerve) is a branch of the pterygopalatine ganglion that carries both general sensory and parasympathetic fibres. It descends through the greater palatine canal, emerges upon the hard palate through

		the greater palatine foramen, and passes forward in a groove in the hard palate towards the incisor teeth. It supplies the gums, the mucous membrane and glands of the hard palate and connects with the terminal filaments of the nasopalatine nerve. Within the pterygopalatine canal, it gives off posterior inferior nasal branches that enter the nasal cavity through openings in the palatine bone, and ramify over the inferior nasal concha and middle and inferior meatuses. As it exits from the canal, a palatine branch is distributed to both surfaces of the soft palate.
4	F	Lingual nerve ➢ The lingual nerve supplies sensory innervations to the tongue. It is a branch of the mandibular nerve (CN V3) division of the trigeminal nerve. It also carries fibers from the facial nerve, which return taste information from the anterior two thirds of the tongue. The lingual nerve supplies general somatic afferent innervation from the mucous membrane of the anterior two-thirds of the tongue. It also carries nerve fibers that are not part of the trigeminal nerve, including the chorda

		tympani nerve of the facial nerve, which provides special sensation (taste) to the anterior 2/3 part of the tongue as well as parasympathetic and sympathetic fibers. ➢ The submandibular ganglion is suspended by two nerve filaments from the lingual nerve. The lingual nerve lies at first beneath the lateral pterygoid muscle, medial to and in front of the inferior alveolar nerve, and is occasionally joined to this nerve by a branch which may cross the internal maxillary artery. ➢ The chorda tympani (a branch of the facial nerve, CN VII) joins it at an acute angle here, carrying taste fibers from the anterior two thirds of the tongue and parasympathetic fibers to the ganglion. The nerve then passes between the medial pterygoid muscle and the ramus of the mandible, and crosses obliquely to the side of the tongue over the constrictor pharyngis superior and styloglossus, and then between the hyoglossus and deep part of the submandibular gland; it finally runs from laterally to medially inferiorly crossing the duct of the submandibular gland, and along the

		tongue to its tip becoming the sublingual nerve, lying immediately beneath the mucous membrane. ➢ Dental procedures and in particular the administration of local anaesthetic can cause damage to the lingual nerve leading to lingual nerve neuropathy.

5	I	Ophthalmic nerve
		➢ The ophthalmic nerve (V1) is one of the three branches of the trigeminal nerve, the fifth cranial nerve. The ophthalmic nerve carries only sensory fibers. The branches of the ophthalmic nerve are
		➢ Nasociliary nerve
		    ➢ sensory root of ciliary ganglion
		    ➢ posterior ethmoidal nerve
		    ➢ long ciliary nerve
		    ➢ infratrochlear nerve
		    ➢ anterior ethmoidal nerve
		➢ lacrimal nerve
		➢ frontal nerve
		    ➢ supratrochlear nerve
		    ➢ supraorbital nerve
		➢ The ophthalmic nerve supplies branches to the cornea, ciliary body, and iris; to the lacrimal gland and

		conjunctiva; to the part of the mucous membrane of the nasal cavity; and to the skin of the eyelids, eyebrow, forehead and nose. It is the smallest of the three divisions of the trigeminal, and arises from the upper part of the trigeminal ganglion as a short, flattened band, about 2.5 cm. long, which passes forward along the lateral wall of the cavernous sinus, below the oculomotor and trochlear nerves; just before entering the orbit, through the superior orbital fissure, it divides into three branches, lacrimal, frontal, and nasociliary. ➢ The frontal branch passes through the orbit superiorly, reenters the frontal bone briefly before exiting above the orbit through the supraorbital foramen and the supratrochlear notch to provide sensory innervation for the skin of the forehead and scalp. ➢ The lacrimal nerve passes through the orbit superiorly to innervate the lacrimal gland. ➢ The nasociliary branch gives off several sensory branches to the orbit and then continues out through the anterior

		ethmoidal foramen, where it enters the nasal cavity and provides innervation for much of the anterior nasal mucosa. It also gives off a branch which exits through the nasal bones to form the external nasal branch. ➢ The ophthalmic nerve is joined by filaments from the cavernous plexus of the sympathetic, and communicates with the oculomotor, trochlear, and abducent nerves; it gives off a recurrent (meningeal) filament which passes between the layers of the tentorium.
6	M	Tensor tympani myoclonus ➢ Tinnitus is a common complaint. It is frequently brushed off as an untreatable symptom. However, taking a careful history and performing an examination will reveal reversible causes in a substantial subgroup of presenting patients. ➢ Key features of tinnitus include unilateral or bilateral, objective or subjective, pulsed or continuous. Examination should focus on any anatomical feature that can impede sound perception pathways. Pure tone audiogram and tympanometry should

		be performed as a bare minimum. ➢ Tensor tympani myoclonus presents as a drum beat or clicking that is made worse in loud noise (unlike normal tinnitus). It can also be objective with the observer hearing the clicks. ➢ Tympanometry often shows an unstable base line. This can often be a pre–cursor to multiple sclerosis and imaging is recommended. ➢ Treatments include anti epileptic medications and surgery to divide the muscle. Stapedius myoclonus presents similarly but does not show any tympanic membrane movement.
7	F	Glomus tympanicum ➢ Glomus tumours are benign growths of the baroreceptor cells in the middle ear. These baroreceptors are important to help equalise pressure in the middle ear. ➢ Tumours are vascular and present with pulsatile tinnitus. As they grow in the middle ear their pulsations impede sound transference and therefore produce a conductive hearing loss. ➢ Glomus jugulare tumours start at the jugular bulb and grow superiorly to affect the middle ear and mastoid. Glomus tympanicum grows from the

		middle ear into the mastoid and brain. A combination, i.e. glomus jugulotympanicum, may occur. Since this patient has no tumour inferiorly at the jugular bulb it is more likely to be tympanicum. ➢ Treatment includes embolisation and surgical excision. A small proportion of this patient group secretes vasoactive hormones and urine should be tested for vanillylmandelic acid. MRI of the lesion often shows a heterogenous tumour described as salt and pepper.
8	I	Patulous Eustachian tube ➢ Patulous Eustachian tube occurs after significant weight loss, in patients with low BMI or following mucosal atrophy. Sound is transmitted from the nasal cavity to the ear more easily through a wide open Eustachian tube. ➢ Symptoms tend to be unilateral and exacerbated by closing the mouth and the contralateral nostril and asking the patient to breathe deeply. When a patient with this condition has a blocked nose air flows through the mouth and bypasses the Eustachian tube orifice reducing tinnitus. An echoing of one's own voice is associated with patulous Eustachian

		tube but autophony or the loud perception of one's own voice is associated with superior semicircular canal dehiscence. ➢ There are generally no agreed treatments for patulous Eustachian tube. There are case reports of injecting fat or collagen around the Eustachian tube orifice as well as reducing the lumen on the middle ear side. ➢ Superior Semicircular canal dehiscence can be diagnosed by history, visual evoked myogenic potentials and CT scan.
9	J	Spontaneous otoacoustic emissions (OAE) ➢ Outer hair cells help amplify sound to the inner hair cells, which are the sound receptors. Outer hair cells are found in a ratio of 3:1 to inner hair cells. ➢ Otoacoustic emissions are the sounds of the outer hair cells. There are two main types, spontaneous and evoked Spontaneous OAE need no sound stimulus and evoked need sound impulses. The neonatal screening programmes use evoked OAE and to prove a normal sound transference and cochlea function.

		➢ Spontaneous OAE are so quiet that they usually require a powerful microphone to detect them. Rarely, they can be high level. Spontaneous otoacoustic emissions are normal and present in those with tinnitus and people with no hearing difficulty. However, on rare occasions the source of tinnitus has been found to be high-level spontaneous otoacoustic emissions. Interestingly, these are frequently heard by observers but rarely by the patient. ➢ No treatment is necessary other than reassurance.
10	N	Venous malformation ➢ Vascular lesions can be separated into haemangiomas and vascular malformations. ➢ Haemangiomas are usually not present at birth and present in infancy. They grow rapidly, out of proportion of the child's growth. They then involute slowly over the next few years leaving either no sign or a hypopigmented region of skin. When they are present in the airway the patient may need intervention. This can include surgical excision, temporary surgical bypass (tracheostomy) or intravenous beta

		blockers. ➢ Vascular malformations are always present at birth, although they may not be noted until childhood or adulthood depending on their location. They can occur in any vascular structure and are subdivided into groups according which vessel is predominantly affected (lymphangioma, arterial malformation, venous malformation, arteriovenous malformation). ➢ Venous malformations are the most common of all vascular anomalies and are characterised by flat endothelium, slow turnover, dysplastic walls and thin basement membranes. They grow slowly with the patient during childhood and adolescences. They can expand thereafter after injury or during certain hormonal states like pregnancy. Venous malformations are slow flow vascular anomalies. When they are situated around the ear or cochlear nerve they produce a unilateral pulsatile tinnitus that reduces on Valsalva and compression of the jugular bulb. ➢ Treatment can be conservative or interventional. Embolisation and surgical excision have both been

		attempted with varying results.
11	F	T2N1M0 ➢ Staging systems such as the TNM scoring system are largely clinical, based on the best possible estimate of the extent of disease before treatment. It categorises the size and spread of the cancer. The assessment of the primary tumour is based on inspection and palpation when possible and by flexible nasoendoscopy. ➢ The tumour should be confirmed histologically and other pathological data obtained on FNA/biopsy may be included. Head and neck MRI or CT should be performed prior to therapy to supplement staging accuracy. ➢ Once TNM has been done the disease can be staged to help with treatment and prognosis. Stage 1 disease is T1 and T2 with N0, T3 and N1 instantly becomes Stage 2, T4 and N2 becomes Stage 3. Stage 1 disease is normally dealt with using single treatment (surgery or radiotherapy) whereas Stage 2 and 3 need multimodal treatment.
12	A	T1N0M0 ➢ T1 tumours are limited to a sub-site and have been conventionally treated

		with radiotherapy, but with the advent of transoral laser they can be now be surgically treated as well.
13	J	T4N2M1 ➢ This is stage 3 disease. Markers of prognosis include extracapsular spread of the tumour from the lymph node capsule, polynodal involvement and poorly differentiated tumour.
14	L	Rhinitis medicamentosa ➢ The 64-year-old man has rhinitis medicamentosa. The nasal mucosa dilates and constricts in an alternating pattern from one nostril to the other. This is regulated by local factors and the autonomic nervous system. When a patient complains of alternating nasal blockage the underlying pathology is mucosal. ➢ Rhinitis medicamentosa is where the lining of the nose becomes engorged and causes nasal obstruction through the prolonged use of nasal vasoconstrictors. There are generally two classes of nasal decongestants sympathomimetics and imidazolines. Sympathomimetics cause release of endogenous noradrenaline through presynaptic sympathetic nerve fibres which binds alpha receptors to cause

		vasoconstriction. Imidazolines directly activate alpha-2 receptors and cause vasoconstriction. ➢ Pathophysiology is most likely due to 'rebound' vasodilatation of the blood vessels within the lining of the nose, mediated via activation of sympathetic beta-receptors and reduction in natural noradrenaline secondary to a negative feedback loop. ➢ It is therefore recommended that topical nasal decongestants usage is restricted to one week.
15	C	Deviated nasal septum ➢ The man who sustained trauma during the assault is likely to develop a deviated septum. This can occur at the time and may be improved with the manipulation of the nasal bones. If it persists then potentially a septoplasty may be required. ➢ The septum is composed of three main parts; membranous septum, cartilaginous septum and bony septum. The membranous septum extends from the columella and is two layers of mucosa. It lies between the semi-rigid columella and the rigid cartilaginous septum and is thought to act as a shock absorber. The cartilaginous septum is

		made of the quadrilateral cartilage sandwiched between two layers of mucosa. It sits on the anterior nasal spine and maxillary crest. The bony septum is made up of the perpendicular plate of the ethmoid superiorly and the vomer inferiorly. ➢ The anterior 1 cm and superior 1 cm of the septum are important weight bearing structure for the nose and damage to these in surgery can lead to saddling of the nose. ➢ Surgery involves getting beneath a submucoperichondrial plane and restoring the septum to a central position. This is accomplished by a combination of techniques depending on where the deflection is. If the deflection is cartilaginous surgery should concentrate on un-anchoring the cartilage from the maxillary crest and bony septum. If this does not work then scoring the concave surface can help straighten the curve. If this fails then it can be laminated using bony septum. Bony deflections can be resected or rasped down. Care should be taken not to damage the weight bearing regions.
16	G	Nasal polyps

		➢ The 25-year-old has nasal polyps which are non-neoplastic swellings arising from the mucous membranes and paranasal sinuses. ➢ Their aetiology is not fully understood, although studies have postulated allergic, genetic and infective causes. Currently there is no definitive curative therapy. Nasal polyps typically present with symptoms of chronic rhinosinusitis, rhinorrhoea, post-nasal drip and anosmia. ➢ Samter's triad is a medical condition consisting of the triad of asthma, aspirin sensitivity and nasal polyposis. ➢ Treatment includes topical steroids and antihistamines. Oral steroids can be very effective at reducing the size of nasal polyps but the side effects restrict prolonged usage. The use of clarithromycin has recently shown to improve symptoms of rhinosinusitis through immunomodulation. Leukotriene antagonists like monteleukast have been shown to benefit patients with rhinosinusitis and asthma. ➢ Surgery is reserved for patients who have failed medical treatment and include simple nasal polypectomy or

		functional endoscopic sinus surgery for severe nasal polyposis
17	E	Foreign body ➢ Foreign bodies are frequently inserted into the nostrils by children and adults with learning difficulties. A degree of manual dexterity and pincer grip is needed so they are rarely seen in children below the age of 2. The commonest presentation is unilateral fetid discharge. The ensuing unilateral vestibulitis is specific to the paediatric group and is almost pathognomonic. ➢ The commonest positions for a foreign body are the floor of the nose and anterior to the middle turbinate. The foreign body even if inert causes pressure necrosis through local tissue inflammation. Corrosive foreign bodies such as button batteries can cause severe anatomical damage if left in for hours and must be removed as a matter of urgency. ➢ The key to diagnosis is a high degree of suspicion and a cooperative child. It is best to remove the foreign body in the child without having to resort to general anaesthesia. This requires a paediatric friendly room, good nursing and informed parents. Often the best

		chance is the first attempt after which the child will become difficult to keep still. ➢ A few positions described include lying in a bed with a blanket tightly rapped around the patient, sitting inbetween a parents legs with the one arm across the chest and arms and the other across the forehead. A blunt probe is used to get behind the foreign body in order to rake it out. If this fails then one should proceed to examination under general anaesthesia.
18	A	Avoid contact sport ➢ Mononucleosis is a contagious disease that is most often caused by the Epstein–Barr virus (EBV) but can also be caused by other viruses such as cytomegalovirus. The incubation period of the EB virus is 2- to 8-weeks followed by an acute phase of 2- to 8-weeks. During this time, the virus can shed intermittently. ➢ Spleen enlargement and rupture is the most serious complication, occurring in approximately 0.5% of individuals, 90% of whom are men; autoimmune haemolytic anaemia affects an estimated 1% to 3% of individuals and thrombocytopenia may occur in up to

		50% of cases. ➢ Active mononucleosis can be detected with a Paul Bunnell, Monospot-test, or Ig M to EBV. ➢ It presents in young adults with severe sore throat. Examination often shows a confluent exudate over the tonsils. Recovery can take weeks. ➢ Treatment is supportive with analgesia and information about lifestyle modifications such as above.
19	I	Patient to inform the driver licensing authority, e.g. in the UK, the Driver and Vehicle Licensing Agency ➢ An AHI greater than 40 suggest severe obstructive sleep apnoea and Group 2 drivers (e.g. heavy good vehicles) guidelines state driving must cease until satisfactory control of symptoms has been attained, with ongoing compliance with treatment, confirmed by consultant/specialist opinion. ➢ Initially it is the responsibility of the patient to inform the DVLA and the doctor must make this clear. If the patient fails to do so then it is the doctor responsible to inform the DVLA. ➢ Other ENT conditions that require DVLA notification include acoustic neuroma, deafness, labyrinthitis,

		Ménière's, and Obstructive sleep apnoea. ➢ These conditions do not necessarily preclude driving but the DVLA has to assess driving safety. When the condition is well controlled then driving can resume.
20	H	Note and adhere to the expiry dates on food ➢ Anosmia is a common symptom and can be congenital (Kallmann syndrome) or acquired. When acquired the pathology can be conductive (as in particles unable to get to olfactory niche due to nasal blockage) or sensorineural (following viral neuronitis). Sensorineural can come on rapidly and patients often feel more debilitated than with conductive anosmia which comes on slowly. Conductive causes (e.g. rhinitis or polyps) are reversible whereas sensorineural causes are generally not. ➢ Treatments for conductive causes include steroids and surgery to improve the anatomical pathways to the olfactory niche. Patients with anosmia should be counselled on the dangers of food expiration and early warning systems for gas leaks. They should be advised to get a smoke

		alarm and change gas cookers to electric ones.
21	D	Do not immerse in water ➢ Wound healing can take weeks to years and progresses in three distinct phases. However, the process is not linear can progress back and forth from the same stage depending on local and external factors. ➢ The first phase is inflammatory and normally lasts 0–10 days (Median 1 day). During this phase bleeding occurs into the wound bed and a haematoma is formed. This is followed by haemostasis. Once haemostasis has been successfully completed the blood vessels dilate to allow essential cells and mediators into the wound bed (white cells, growth factors, enzymes and nutrients). During this period inflammation and erythema are seen around the wound edges. The main cells at work here are the neutrophils and macrophages. ➢ The following stage is proliferation when the wound is rebuilt. This occurs by secretion of fibroblasts into the wound. These cells help built the granulation tissue that will populate the wound and bring the edges

		together. This process can take up to day 30 but median time shows it's completed by day 10. ➢ Maturation is the final step and can take up to 100 days. This involves remodelling the collagen from type 3 to type 1. ➢ Dressings are used to absorb secretions from the wound in most cases, however, in awkward positions or poorly healing wounds a cellulose based dressing can be used to aid healing. General advice for wound care is to allow at least 3 days before immersing in water so as to allow the edges to adhere together.
22	L	Reduced salt in diet ➢ This patient has Ménière's disease. The condition is a triad of episodic vertigo, tinnitus, and low frequency hearing loss. It is a rare condition and must have all three symptoms to be diagnosed. ➢ The underlying pathophysiology is not fully understood but there is always endolymphatic hydrops. ➢ Diagnosis is mostly clinical but can be assisted with electrocochleography which shows a summating potential to action

		potential ratio of 0.5. ➢ Treatment for this condition includes reduction of salt in the diet and regular betahistine (vasodilator). ➢ When this fails the options include intratympanic steroids, intratympanic gentamicin and saccus decompression. The intratympanic gentamicin has a risk of hearing loss, although aminoglycosides are more toxic to the labyrinth compared to the cochlea. The saccus decompression surgery also has a risk of hearing loss and this is operator dependent. ➢ The management of this condition also involves life style changes such as reduction of salt in the diet, avoiding chocolate and caffeine drinks.
23	J	T1 ➢ It is important to know the basic anatomical derivation of the cervical and brachial plexuses. The intrinsic muscles of the hands appear to be affected and these muscles are supplied by T1. The ulnar nerve delivers this T1 nerve to the interossei of the hand. ➢ The motor function of T1 is checked by

		asking a patient to abduct all fingers against force. Sensory innervation of T1 is on the medial surface of the upper arm. ➢ As this nerve is closest, of the brachial plexus nerves, to the lung pleura it is at greatest risk from upper lobe lung cancers. Compromise of the nerve due to lung cancer is known as Lambert–Eaton syndrome.
24	L	T1–L2 (Sympathetic chain) ➢ All sympathetic efferents emerge from T1–L2 levels of the spinal cord. They integrate with each other in the paraspinal ganglia and then journey to their target. Sympathetic nerves from T1–T4 form the superior cervical ganglion which is found around the C3 vertebra. They travel along the carotid to the face where they supply the head and neck. ➢ The cervical sympathetic trunk runs up the neck on the fascia that lies in front of the longus muscles. At the top of the trunk is the thickening representing the largest cervical ganglion (superior), adjacent to C6. The inferior ganglion may be fused with the first thoracic ganglion to form a single structure, the stellate ganglion, adjacent to C7.

		➢ Postganglionic axons projects to target: (heart, head, neck) via 'hitchhiking' on the carotid arteries. They supply the heart, lower neck, arm, posterior cranial arteries. ➢ Nerves emerging from cervical sympathetic ganglia also contribute to the cardiac plexus, among other things. ➢ Interruption of the upper sympathetic chain leads of Horner's syndrome: dropping of upper eyelid, anhydrosis miosis and enophthalmos. The droopy eyelid is due to loss of sympathetic innervation to the levator palpebrae superioris muscle, which is also innervated by the oculomotor nerve. Sympathetic overactivity is seen in Grave's disease of the thyroid gland and this causes exophthalmos because of increased contraction of the levator palpebrae superioris muscle.
25	E	C5 ➢ The deltoid area is supplied by C5 as is shoulder abduction. The brachial plexus is a somatic nerve plexus formed by intercommunications among the ventral rami (roots) of the lower four cervical nerves (C5–C8) and the first thoracic nerve (T1).

		➢ The roots of the brachial plexus emerge from the transverse processes of their respective cervical vertebra and join together to become trunks. The trunks run inbetween the anterior and middle scalene muscles. The divisions are lateral to the first rib and posterior to the axillary artery. These give rise to cords which are named in relation to the axillary artery.
26	J	T1 ➢ The medial aspect of the forearm is supplied by T1 mainly, with a small contribution from C8. ➢ Other important nerves in the neck include the greater auricular, spinal accessory, ansa cervicalis and the phrenic nerve. ➢ The greater auricular nerve is a superior branch of the cervical plexus. It innervates the skin over the parotid, the mastoid and the ear lobe. It is derived from C2 and C3. It traverses over sternocleidomastoid and is of importance as it can be used as a cable nerve graft (for facial nerve paralysis) or to directly reinnervate the larynx, but also as it is an important landmark for the spinal accessory nerve. ➢ The spinal accessory nerve is

		composed of a cranial portion and a cervical portion. The cranial portion, which originates from nucleus ambiguous runs most of its course in accessory to the vagus nerve (hence the name) and innervates pharyngeal muscles (levator veli palatini). The cervical portion enters the skull via the foramen magnum and exits via the jugular foramen. It runs anterior to the internal jugular vein and then medial to the digastric muscle before it heads for sternocleidomastoid. It pierces and innervates this muscle. It exits posteriorly at Erb's point (1cm superior to the point where the greater auricular crosses the posterior margin of sternocleidomastoid). The other marker for this nerve is from the junction of the upper third and lower two thirds of the posterior edge of the sternocleidomastoid to the junction of the lower third and upper two thirds of the anterior border of the trapezius muscle.
27	I	Long Thoracic nerve of Bell ➢ The long thoracic nerve of Bell supplies the serratus anterior muscle (hence it is sometimes referred to as nerve to serratus anterior). This nerve

		characteristically arises by three roots from the fifth, sixth, and seventh cervical nerves (C5–C7) but the root from C7 is not always present. Damage to this nerve causing winging of the scapula. ➢ The ansa cervicalis is another nerve of importance. This is in fact is the ring of the neck and receives nerve inputs from hypoglossal nerve, C1, C2 and C3. It supplies all the strap muscles other than thyrohyoid which is innervated by the ventral root of C1. The ansa can be used to reinnervate the larynx if necessary. It runs anterior to the jugular vein and is found in the carotid sheath. ➢ The phrenic nerves originate from C3, 4 and 5. It innervates the diaphragm. Its position in the neck is noted as it is the only nerve that runs mediolaterally on the anterior scalene.
28	J	Oral Penicillin V ➢ Penicillins block cell wall synthesis by inhibition of peptidoglycan cross linkage. This is achieved by binding penicillin binding proteins, blocking transpeptidase and activation of autolytic enzymes. It is used for gram positive organisms as it is not taken up by cell membrane of gram

		negative organisms. ➢ Rods are rare cause of ENT disease but include clostridium, anthrax, listeria and diphtheria. ➢ The cocci are added to catalase and if they clump into clusters they're staphylococcus, but if they gather into chains they are streptococcus. These streptococci are added to a blood mixture and their ability to haemolyse is noted. Complete haemolysis (clear colour) indicates beta haemolytic streptococci (Strep pyogenes which is Group A or Strep agalactiae which is Group B). Partial haemolysis (green colour) indicates Strep pneumoniae (capsule) or Viridans streptococci (no capsule). ➢ In an uncomplicated case of bacterial tonsillitis Penicillin V is the antibiotic of choice, as usually in bacterial infections the organism of concern is the Lancefield's Group A beta-haemolytic streptococcus which is still susceptible to penicillin.
29	E	Oral amoxicillin ➢ Amoxicillin is a moderate-spectrum, bacteriolytic, β-lactam antibiotic used to treat bacterial infections caused by susceptible microorganisms. It is usually the drug of choice within the

		class because it is better absorbed, following oral administration, than other β-lactam antibiotics. Amoxicillin is one of the most common antibiotics prescribed for children. ➢ However, it is important to avoid the use of synthetic ampicillin (and amoxicillin) in glandular fever because it increases the occurrence of a macular rash. This has lead to litigation as rarely it can be permanent. Penicillin V is the treatment of choice. ➢ Amoxicillin is susceptible to degradation by β-lactamase-producing bacteria, which are resistant to a broad spectrum of β-lactam antibiotics, such as penicillin. For this reason, it is often combined with clavulanic acid, a β-lactamase inhibitor, and marketed under one name Co-amoxiclav. This increases effectiveness by reducing its susceptibility to β-lactamase resistance.
30	D	IV Metronidazole ➢ Metronidazole is usually used in combination in para tonsillar abscesses due to the anaerobic cover it provides. Metronidazole works by releasing free radicals within the bacterium that

		damages DNA. It cannot be used in pregnancy or when trying to conceive. It causes a disulfiram type reaction with alcohol and advice must be given. ➢ Metronidazole is a nitroimidazole antibiotic medication used particularly for anaerobic bacteria and protozoa. It is an antibiotic, amoebicide, and antiprotozoal and is the drug of choice for first episodes of mild-to-moderate Clostridium difficile infection. ➢ Metronidazole is taken up by diffusion and is selectively absorbed by anaerobic bacteria and sensitive protozoa. It is non-enzymatically reduced by reacting with reduced ferredoxin, which is generated by pyruvate oxidoreductase. Many of the reduced nitroso intermediates will form sulfonamides and thioether linkages with cysteine bearing enzymes deactivating these critical enzymes. As many as 150 separate enzymes are affected. In addition or alternatively, the metronidazole metabolites are taken up into bacterial DNA, and form unstable molecules. This function only occurs when metronidazole is partially reduced, and because this reduction usually happens only in anaerobic cells,

		it has relatively little effect upon human cells or aerobic bacteria.
31	B	IV Cefotaxime ➢ Epiglottitis is a life-threatening condition that is caused by bacterial infection of the epiglottis, aryepiglottis, and arytenoids. It is differentiated from viral croup and foreign body aspiration by the acutely ill appearance of patient. ➢ Epiglottitis is a paediatric emergency. Acute disease generally occurs in children between the ages of 2- and 6-years. Haemophilus influenzae type B causes more than 75% of cases. It is now relatively rare due to the Haemophilus vaccine (HiB). Rarely, other bacterial causes include beta-haemolytic streptococci, staphylococci and pneumococci. ➢ Second-and-third-generation cephalosporins, such as ceftriaxone, cefuroxime or cefotaxime, are the antibiotics of choice for acute epiglottitis because of the high prevalence of ampicillin-resistant strains of HIB.
32	B	Respiratory alkalosis ➢ In the first scenario the girl has a history suggestive of hyperventilation

			syndrome. This causes a reduction in the PCO2. The loss of this respiratory acid leads to an alkalosis. As a result, using the Henderson Hasselbalch equation, excess bicarbonate in the plasma is converted to carbonic acid and then to carbon dioxide. Although this metabolic compensation does occur, it cannot occur fast enough to neutralise the alkalosis in a rapid onset of hyperventilation. ➢ Alkalosis leads to dissociation of hydrogen ions from albumin. This leaves albumin sites free to associate with ionized calcium. The free ionized calcium fraction is the clinically effective portion and the reduction of this fraction leads to symptoms of hypocalcaemia despite total body calcium being normal. ➢ The hypocalcaemia causes cerebral vasoconstriction and tetany. Carpopedal spasm results with minimal arm compression (Trousseau's sign), and facial nerve activation can occur with tapping over the nerve (Chvostek's sign). It is important to understand the physiology of calcium as surgery to the thyroid or parathyroid can lead to calcium dysregulation.

33	F	Diabetic ketoacidosis ➢ The 25-year-old man has diabetic ketoacidosis. It may be defined by serum bicarbonate of 16 mmol/L, ketonaemia, hyperglycaemia, and mental impairment. ➢ His arterial blood gas would show a severe metabolic acidosis with a low carbon dioxide secondary to increased respiratory drive from the acidosis. ➢ Acidosis is a late sign of sepsis and is a poor prognostic indicator. ➢ It should be investigated by a blood gas and corrected with aggressive fluid therapy. Treatment involves slow rehydration to prevent central pontine myelinolysis.
34	D	Respiratory and metabolic acidosis ➢ The 72-year-old male has suffered a loss of cardiac output and ventilatory failure. He is being inadequately ventilated due to the bag and mask. An arterial blood gas would reveal a severe metabolic acidosis as a result of loss of cardiac output combined with poor tissue perfusion. ➢ Hypoxia and hypercarbia result from poor ventilation. Hypercarbia would exacerbate the acidosis. The overall result is a combined respiratory and

		metabolic acidosis.
35	K	200 mls ➢ It is important to understand how to calculate drug doses as you frequently have to calculate local anaesthetic and injectable drug doses. To calculate a maximum safe dose it is important to know the maximum allowed dose per weight. ➢ Unfortunately, this is normally in milligrams of drug per kilograms patient weight. Drugs are normally provided in percentage of drug per mL or concentration. And therefore a conversion calculation is needed. ➢ 1% of a solution has 10 mg of the drug per mL. Equally a 1:100 solution of adrenaline has 1 mL of adrenaline in 100 mL of solution (or 0.01 mL of adrenaline in 1 mL of solution) or 10 mg of adrenaline in 1 mL of solution. Topical adrenaline is normally used in 1:1000 (1 mg). This can be diluted to 1:100,000 by adding 1 mL of 1:1000 to a 100 mL. Within the 100 mL there will actually by 0.01 mL of adrenaline. 1:200,000 is equivalent to 1 mL of adrenaline in 200,000 mL of solution or 0.01 mL of adrenaline in 200 mL of solution.

		➢ Therefore, the addition of 200 mL of saline can be added to 1:1000 adrenaline to make 1:200,000. This dose is commonly used as an adjunct to bupivacaine in local anaesthetics. ➢ The simplification is below: Adding 100 mL to 1:1000 will make 1:100,000 Further dilution to 1:200,000 would require another 100 mls. Therefore the total amount is 200 mL
36	G	20 mL ➢ Lidocaine is a very commonly used local anaesthetic. It acts on sodium channels of nerves and blocks nerve conduction. The maximum dose is 3 mg of lidocaine per kilogram weight of patient. This increases to 7 mg/kg if adrenaline is used as an adjunct. ➢ 1% lidocaine is equivalent to 10 mg of lidocaine in 1 mL of solution. For an average 70 kg man the maximum dose of lidocaine without adrenaline is 210 mg (70 kg x 3 mg). If 10 mg are in every 1 mL, then 21 mL of 1%lidocaine is needed to make 210 mg of lidocaine. ➢ If 0.5% lidocaine is used then 5 mg lidocaine is in every 1 mL of solution and 42 mL of solution will be needed to make the maximum dose of 210 mg. And if 2% lidocaine is used than 10.5

<table>
<tr><td></td><td></td><td>mL lidocaine will be make up the maximum dose.

Safe dose of lignocaine without adrenaline is 3 mg/kg
Therefore a 70 kg man requires 210 mg of lignocaine
1% lignocaine has 10 mg/mL lignocaine
Hence 210 mg of lignocaine would be in 21 mL of 1% lignocaine
The closest answer given in the options is 20 mL</td></tr>
<tr><td>37</td><td>C</td><td>4 mls
➢ Cocaine is commonly used as a topical anaesthetic in the nose in the Moffatt's solution (classically 2 mL 5% cocaine, 1 mL 1:1000 adrenaline and 2 mL 8.4% bicarbonate).
➢ This is made up by the ENT surgeon prior to surgery and it is essential to understand drug calculations for this reason.
➢ The maximum dose of cocaine is 3 mg of drug for every kilogram of the patient. For an average 70 kg man that would be equivalent to 210 mg of cocaine. 1 mg of cocaine contains 10 mg in 1 mL of solution and therefore 10% cocaine contains 100 mg in 1 mL. 2 mL of 10% therefore equates to 200</td></tr>
</table>

		mg cocaine. However for a 50 kg woman using the same dose calculation we can see the maximum dose is 150 mg and therefore 2 mL of 10% cocaine used in a standard Moffat's solution would be an overdose. ➢ In this question the following calculation provides the answer. 1% cocaine contadins 10 mg/ml 5% cocaine contains 50 mg/ml Therefore 4 mL of 5% cocaine would contain 200 mg of cocaine
38	F	10 mL ➢ This dose calculation is the most difficult. There are a few concepts that will make things easier. 1:100 adrenaline is the equivalent to 1%. 100% of any drug is equivalent to 1000 mg in 1 mL of solution. ➢ Using a similar calculation technique 1:80,000 is equivalent to 0.00125% of adrenaline (1/80,000 x 100 = 1/800). If 100% is 1000 mg then 0.00125% is 0.0125 mg of adrenaline in 1 mL (1000 mg/100 x 0.00125 = 10 x 0.00125 = 0.0125 mg). Therefore 10 mL of this solution will provide 0.125 mg of adrenaline total dose. Below is a simplification.

		10 mg/mL = 1:100 Therefore 0.01 mg/mL = 100,000 (simply move the decimal three places to the left because it is a dilution process) This means that 0.0125 mg/mL = 1:80,000 (because this is a more concentrated solution you have to multiple by 0.01 by 100,000/80,000 Therefore 10 mL of solution would contain 0.125 mg (simply move the decimal one place to the right)
39	C	Aphthous ulcer ➢ Aphthous ulcers are painful, shallow ulcers on the tongue or mucosal surface of the mouth. The ulcer starts as a small vesicle which then breaks down. Healing occurs without scarring. ➢ The exact cause of many aphthous ulcers is unknown but citrus fruits, physical trauma, stress, lack of sleep, sudden weight loss, food allergies, immune system reactions and deficiencies in vitamin B12, iron, and folic acid may contribute to their development. ➢ There appears to be a familial tendency. It is slightly more common in women than men and is most frequent in childhood and adolescence.

		➢ They are normally 2–4 mm in size, round or ovoid in shape with a yellow base that becomes gray as it heals. There is often an erythematous halo surrounding the ulcer. ➢ They tend to last 10–14 days and occur on non- keratinized squamous epithelium, so the hard palate is spared. ➢ Treatment is supportive with topical barrier creams that contain analgesic properties.
40	I	Squamous papilloma ➢ Oral squamous papillomas make up 3% of all oral biopsied lesions. They are induced by human papilloma viruses 6 and 11, which have been linked to malignancy. ➢ HPV is a DNA virus, of the papovavirus group, capable of integrating its DNA into the host genome. All HPV viruses are infectious; however, squamous papilloma has a low virulence rate. ➢ Nasal, paranasal and laryngeal papillomata are identical to oropharyngeal warts histologically, but they behave differently. Oral papillomata have lower recurrence rates and tend to occur in isolation, not in clusters. They also stop growing

		sooner than their head and neck counterparts. ➢ The condition is more common between the ages of 30 and 50. There is no sex predilection. Any surface can be affected but the tongue is the most common. The typical lesion is a soft, pedunculated mass with numerous fingers like surface projections. The disease in children resolves spontaneously in 2/3 of patients. Surgery has low recurrence rates but must include removal of the base.
41	A	Actinomycosis ➢ Actinomycosis is an infectious bacterial disease caused by Actinomyces anaerobic gram-positive branching filamentous rod shaped bacteria such as Actinomyces israelii. ➢ The disease is characterised by the formation of painful abscesses in the mouth, lungs or gastrointestinal tract. Actinomyces abscesses grow larger as the disease progresses, often over months. The purulent leakage via the sinus cavities contains 'sulphur granules,' which only actually resemble such particles. ➢ Cervicofacial actinomycosis tends to follow after oral surgery when the

		bacteria leaks from tonsils/teeth into the gum tissues. Initial symptoms are pains and swelling along the alveolar ridge and soft tissues of the perimandibular regions. There is direct spread into adjacent tissues and enlargement of lymph nodes. Subsequent areas of swelling occur and turn into sinuses and fistulae that disease sulphur granules. Bone involvement is a characteristic feature and results in periostitis and osteomyelitis. If the maxillary bone is involves cranial nerve palsies may develop.
42	J	Trotter's syndrome ➢ The sinus of Morgagni is the space between the superior constrictor inferiorly and the skull base superiorly. It is lined by nasopharyngeal mucosa anteriorly and the pharyngobasilar membrane posteriorly. Since the superior constrictor only touches the skull base in the midline, the spaces laterally are just two fascial planes. On the posterior side is foramen ovale and mandibular division of the trigeminal nerve. On the anterior side is the fossa of Rosenmüller, and the eustachian tube orifice.

		➢ The syndrome is due to malignant nasopharyngeal carcinoma invading through the sinus of Morgagni. In the syndrome pain is experienced in the jaw and tongue on the side of the tumour. The palate is often deviated and there is unilateral conductive deafness. There is restricted mobility of the internal pterygoid and palatine muscles. It is an ominous presentation, which can masquerade as dental or masticatory pain.
43	A	Alexander's law ➢ Alexander's law states that in individuals with nystagmus, the amplitude of the nystagmus increases when the eye moves in the direction of the fast phase (saccade). ➢ It is manifested during spontaneous nystagmus in a patient with a vestibular lesion. The nystagmus becomes more intense when the patient looks in the direction of the quick phase. ➢ Working example: Disease of the vestibular apparatus can be due to over activity (during active labyrinthitis) or secondary to paralysis (following severe labyrinthitis). Movement of your head to the right

		causes the right vestibular apparatus to fire more than the left. This causes your eyes to drift to the left and thereby allowing optical fixation (this is a slow movement). When the right vestibular apparatus is activated by infection it erroneously causes your eyes to drift to the left (slowly). Your brain realises this is incorrect and quickly readjusts your gaze to the centre (by rapid eye movement to the right). This is the basis of nystagmus. ➢ During an active infection of the right vestibular apparatus there is consistent drive to move your eyes to the left. By moving your eyes to the right (or in the direction of the fast phase of nystagmus in this case) you will further combat this impulse and aggravate the nystagmus. Hence people with right-sided labyrinthitis prefer to look to the left.
44	K	Tullio's phenomena ➢ The inner ear works by movement of hair cell inducing action potential, This may be small vibrations of air (sound) causing the perilymph to move over the hair cell attached to a tectorial membrane and causing it to become activated, or with head movement

		causing movement of perilymph over hair cell in the semicircular canals. ➢ The cochlea and vestibular apparatus are separated from each other so activation of one does not necessarily cause activation of the other. ➢ The Tullio phenomenon is a syndrome in which acoustic stimulation produces symptoms and signs of vestibular activation (i.e. sound-induced vertigo, dizziness, nausea and/nystagmus). Tullio's occurs mainly in five ear conditions: Superior canal dehiscence, perilymph fistula, Ménière's syndrome, post fenestration surgery and vestibulofibrosis. It can also be present in congenital syphilis. ➢ In essence sound vibrations are causing activation of hair cells in the semicircular canal. Surgical repair of the defect leads to resolution of symptoms.
45	F	Grisel syndrome ➢ This is also known as nasopharyngeal torticollis and is due to non-traumatic subluxation of the atlantoaxial joint. The condition is also associated with infection such adenotonsillitis, parotiditis and cervical abscesses. ➢ Sudeck's sign may also be present,

		which is displacement of the spine of the axis. It may be due to over distention of the joint ligaments, rupture of the transverse ligament, excessive passive rotation during the general anaesthesia. ➢ However other theories suggest that there is a rich communication between the periodontal venous plexus and the pharyngovertebral veins. Therefore exudates from infection can easily be transported to the spine, leading to inflammation and disarticulation. ➢ Children are more prone to this condition. This may be due to the steep dens-facet angle or due to the rich anastomoses between the head and the spine. ➢ Treatment includes skeletal skull traction to re-align the odontoid peg followed by 3 months of immobilisation. This is usually successful.
46	D	Boyce's sign ➢ This refers to a lump in the neck that gurgles on palpation and is a sign of a pharyngeal pouch. ➢ This is not to be confused with Bryce's sign which is gurgling in the neck secondary to a laryngocoele.

			➢ It may be worth noting that Boyle's ligament is the anterior commissure ligament connecting the vocal cord to the larynx and represents the path of least resistance for the spread of squamous cell carcinoma through the thyroid cartilage. ➢ A laryngocoele is a dilatation of the laryngeal vestibule. It is commonly seen in men in their fifth decade and is more common in professional blowers (glass blowers, wind instrument players etc). ➢ The laryngeal vestibule is the air filled gap between the true and false vocal cords. It is a vestigial remnant of air filled sacs thought to be able to hold large volumes of air for rebreathing during sea diving. In this condition the vestibule enlarges. It is classified as internal if it lies within the thyroid cartilage and external if it pierces the thyrohyoid membrane. External laryngocoeles can change in size during forced expiration against a blockage (playing an instrument) and it is during this manoeuvre that they present as a neck mass. They can become filled with mucous or infected. They rarely occur due to blockage of normal air flows

		from a carcinoma and this must be ruled out if a laryngocoele is diagnosed. ➢ Investigation with T1 weighted MRI is diagnostic. Treatment involves endoscopic or open surgical excision.
47	H	Measles. ➢ The prodromal phase of measles (caused by a single serotype paramyxovirus) is characterised by upper respiratory catarrh and Koplik's spots on the buccal mucosa. This is accompanied by conjunctivitis, otitis media and rhinitis. After 24–48 hours, a maculopapular rash appears on the face and spreads peripherally via the trunk. ➢ The condition last for 7–10 days, following which the fading rash leaves skin staining, brown macules with fine desquamation that can last for up to 3 weeks. ➢ Spread is via airborne droplet transmission for the respiratory tract of patients with active measles. Patients are infectiousness 2 days before symptoms and 4 days after the onset of the rash. Small white spots in the mouth (Koplik's spots) appear within 2 days of the prodromal

		symptoms and last 4 days. ➢ Complications are more common before 5 and after 20-years-old. The most common is pneumonia followed by otitis media. Rare complications include subacute sclerosing panencephalitis and disseminated intravascular coagulation.
48	F	Kawasaki ➢ Kawasaki disease is an acute febrile vasculitic illness of early childhood. The condition is also known as mucocutaneous lymph node syndrome and infantile periarteritis nodosa. ➢ Children with Kawasaki disease presented with fever, rash, conjunctival injection, cervical lymphadenitis, inflammation of the lips and oral cavity, and erythema and edema of the hands and feet. ➢ Intravenous immunoglobulin (IVIG) and aspirin have constituted the mainstays of therapy for Kawasaki disease. Corticosteroids and infliximab have been used in patients with disease refractory to IVIG. ➢ The disease has a 2% mortality which is related to coronary thromboses. 25% of untreated patients develop myocardial complications. There is no

		test for this condition and it is diagnosed on clinical grounds.
49	E	Infectious mononucleosis ➢ Infectious mononucleosis is a self-limiting infection, most often caused by Epstein–Barr virus (EBV). However, approximately 10% of those with IM are not acutely infected with EBV and many of these have symptoms attributable to cytomegalovirus (CMV) infection. ➢ IM is particularly common in adolescents and children. The main symptoms of mononucleosis are a sore throat, fever, fatigue, malaise, pharyngeal inflammation, vomiting, petechiae and loss of appetite. ➢ Common signs include lymphadenopathy, hepatosplenomegaly. Symptomatic treatment is required. ➢ Diagnosis is based on Paul Bunnell or Monospot-tests. ➢ Advice must be given to avoid contact and thus prevent the risk of splenic rupture.
50	K	Scarlet fever ➢ Scarlet fever is a disease caused by exotoxin released from Streptococcus pyogenes. The rash is the most characteristic sign of scarlet fever. ➢ It starts off looking like sunburn with

		tiny bumps and it may itch. The rash usually appears first on the neck and face and then spreads to the chest and back, and subsequently to the rest of the body. Areas of rash usually turn whitish. By the sixth day of the infection, the rash usually fades but the affected skin may peel like sunburn. ➢ Other symptoms include high fever, a reddened sore throat and cervical lymphadenopathy. ➢ Scarlet fever may be prevented by adenotonsillectomy. ➢ Diagnosis is clinical and treatment is supportive with antibiotics.
51	L	Steven–Johnson syndrome ➢ Stevens–Johnson syndrome and toxic epidermal necrolysis are two forms of a life-threatening skin condition, in which cell death causes the epidermis to separate from the dermis. ➢ The syndrome is thought to be a hypersensitivity complex that affects the skin and the mucous membranes. The main cause, as in this case, is a reaction to medication. It may also follow an infections and rarely, cancers. The reaction usually begins with fever, sore throat. ➢ It is commonly misdiagnosed and treated

		with antibiotics. Ulcers and other lesions begin to appear in the mucous membranes, especially in the mouth and lips but also in the genital and anal regions. Those in the mouth are usually extremely painful and best treated with Kenalog in Orabase. Conjunctivitis of the eyes may also occur. ➢ A rash of round lesions may also be present on the face, trunk, arms and legs, and soles of the feet but not the scalp.
52	E	Normal hearing ➢ In the Weber's test a vibrating tuning fork (either 256 or 512 Hz) is placed in the middle of the forehead or the vertex. At less than 256 Hz it is hard to decipher whether the patient perceives sound or the vibration. Any higher than 512 Hz and it doesn't last long enough for those hard of hearing to perceive. ➢ Weber's test works on the premise that conductive hearing loss results in a slight improvement in conductive hearing. Placing the base of the tuning fork on the vertex or incisors makes the test more sensitive. On the whole it picks up conductive losses greater than 10 dB. The patient is asked to report in which ear the sound is heard louder. In a normal patient, the sound is heard

		equally in both ears (no lateralisation) and this can be corroborated by a normal pure tone audiogram. ➢ If it lateralises then this can either represent an ipsilateral conductive hearing loss or a contralateral sensorineural hearing loss.
53	C	Conductive hearing loss left side ➢ Rinne's is usually performed by placing the tuning fork in front of the ear and then on the mastoid. The patient is asked say where the sound is louder. Normally air conduction (in front the ear) is better than bone conduction (behind the ear). This is known as Rinne positive. ➢ The test may become negative if there is a sensorineural hearing loss or if there is a difference in the air bone gap of more than 20 dB when a 512 Hz tuning fork is used. A smaller air bone gap (15 dB) would be detected by a 256 Hz tuning fork. The 512 Hz tuning fork is most commonly used in clinical practice.
54	A	Asterion ➢ Neurootologist use this point to orientate themselves, in order to plan safe entry into the skull for acoustic neuromas. It is sometimes called the

			‘Mercedes point’ because of its resemblance to the Mercedes–Benz logo. ➢ It is the confluence point of three suture lines: lambdoid, parieto mastoid, and occipitomastoid. It is also the point where three bones meet: the mastoid part of the temporal bone, the parietal and occipital bones. ➢ There are three main approaches to an acoustic neuroma: Translabyrinthine, retrosigmoid and middle cranial fossa. ➢ Translab approaches the internal auditory meatus by drilling through the cochlea and semicircular canals. Therefore hearing loss and dysequilibrium are guaranteed. It should be considered for small tumours, mostly in the IAM and where hearing has already been compromised. Since the facial nerve is identified early, damage is unlikely. ➢ The middle cranial fossa approach is good for small tumours, mostly in the internal auditory meatus. The temporal lobe has to be retracted and this can occasionally cause lasting problems with speech. The IAM is approached from above. Since the facial nerve is the most superior nerve in the IAM it is

		at risk here and often has to be moved out of the way to get to the vestibular schwannoma. This approach is good for hearing preservation. ➢ The retrosigmoid approach is used for large tumours or tumours that are mostly intracranial. Retraction of the cerebellum is necessary to get a good view. This approach has a high rate of neck and head aches.
55	F	Pterion ➢ The pterion is not a single point but an area where the parietal, frontal, squamous part of the temporal bone and the greater wing of the sphenoid meet. ➢ Pterion is derived from the Greek word for wings. It is the weakest part of the skull. It is also the point over which the anterior division of the middle meningeal artery runs. Therefore it is highly prone to fracture and this often leads to tearing of large intracranial blood vessel causing an extradural haematoma. ➢ An extradural haematoma presents with a loss of consciousness and then a lucid interval. This is followed by an expanding haematoma, raising intracranial pressure and further loss of

		consciousness with rapid deterioration in Glasgow Coma Scale. ➢ Treatment is urgent surgica evacuation via a burr hole. Small haematomas can be managed conservatively with osmotic diuretics and hyperventilation.
56	H	Spine of Henle ➢ Spine of Henle is a small bony prominence anterior to the supramastoid pit at the posterosuperior margin of the bony external ear canal. It is an important surgical landmark during cortical mastoidectomy. Macewen's triangle forms the boundaries of the mastoid exploration. ➢ Using a post auricular approach, in an incision is made half a centimetre posterior to the post auricular sulcus in a curvilinear fashion. The ear is pulled laterally and the incision in then progressed through layers until the periosteum is reached. The periosteum is incised in a cat-flap fashion. The periosteal flap (superiorly based is elevated revealing underlying cortex. This is one of many approaches that get the surgeon to this stage. ➢ Macewen's triangle is an imaginary

		triangle that lies 1.5 cm above the antrum and is used as the surface markings to begin the mastoidectomy. The triangle is made by a line from the temporal line, joining a line that passes along the posterosuperior canal margin (at the Spine of Henle). These two lines are connected by a line drawn perpendicular to the first. The temporal line is made by tracing the zygomatic root posteriorly and is the surface marking of the lowest point of the dura. Therefore, surgery above this area has the risk of intracranial breach. Macewen's triangle lies posterosuperior to the external auditory canal.
57	C	Inion ➢ This is the most prominent projection of the occipital at the posteroinferior part of the skull where ligamentum nuchae and trapezius muscle attaches. It is sometimes loosely called the external occipital protuberance. ➢ The nasion is the junction of the frontal bone and the nasal bones. ➢ The rhinion is the junction of the nasal bones and upper lateral cartilage. ➢ Skin begins to thin from the nasion and gets to its thinnest point over the

		rhinion. It again thickens over the cartilaginous dorsum. This is an important fact when dealing with dorsal humps as more cartilage will have to be resected compared to bone. ➢ The nasion is an important facial aesthetic point. If the nasion is set high it gives the appearance of a big/long nose. The nasofrontal angle should approximately be 115–130°. This angle which is calculated from the nasion helps in deciding how much dorsal hump to resect and how much saddling to correct.
58	M	Wegener's ➢ Wegener's granulomatosis is a form of systemic vasculitis that primarily affects the upper and lower respiratory tracts and the kidney. ➢ The most common presenting symptoms include persistent rhinorrhoea, purulent/bloody nasal discharge and sinus pain. Kidney involvement manifests with acute renal failure. Other organ systems involved include joints, eyes, ears, skin, nervous system and the heart. ➢ Wegener's granulomatosis is considered to be an 'autoimmune' disease mediated either by cellular

		immune mechanisms or by immune complex deposition. ➢ The disease demonstrates a 2:1 male predominance, and the mean age of onset is 40 years. ➢ Common presenting symptoms include headache, sinusitis, rhinorrhea, otitis media, fever, and arthralgias. The sinus cavities and kidneys are involved in over 90% of patients. Pulmonary manifestations include cough, pleuritic chest pain, haemoptysis, and nodular or cavitary infiltrates on chest radiograph. Approximately 50% of patients have ocular findings of conjunctivitis, iritis, or scleritis, and dermatologic findings of necrotic ulcerations, vesicles, or petechiae.
59	J	Sarcoidosis ➢ Sarcoidosis is a systemic condition involving a type IV hypersensitivity reaction. It mainly affects the lungs but also has extrapulmonary manifestations such as lupus pernio of the nose, parotitis and supraglottic granulomatous lesions. ➢ Lupus pernio is a chronic papulonodular eruption which consists of violaceous, indurated papules, nodules, and plaques they may

		become hardened and fibrotic. It is more common in women than in men. Commonly seen around the central face, ears and especially the alar rim of the nose. ➤ Pulmonary lesions in sarcoidosis include bilateral hilar adenopathy and interstitial apical infiltrates. Later stage disease involves advanced fibrosis. Non-caseating granulomata of the lung are typical of sarcoidosis. ➤ Clinically important renal involvement is an occasional problem in sarcoidosis: Hypercalciuria and hypercalcaemia are most often responsible, but granulomatous interstitial nephritis or glomerular disease may be seen on rare occasions. ➤ Diagnosis used to be with the Kveim test, but with the advent of BSE this has fallen out of grace. Now diagnosis involves blood tests for calcium, angiotensin converting enzyme and radiological/histological supporting features. Hypercalcaemia is cause by vitamin D production in activated macrophages.
60	K	Syphilis ➤ Destruction of the vomer and ethmoid bone accounts for a posterior septal

		perforation, and may be due to a syphilitic gumma. ➢ Syphilis is an infectious venereal disease that is transmitted by sexual contact, materno-fetal transmission and blood transfusion of infected products. ➢ It is caused by Treponema Pallidum a motile gram negative spirochaeta that is capable of movement through. The bacterium is seen under dark-field illumination. ➢ The introduction of penicillin in the twentieth century has caused a massive drop in this disease which has been a cause of great morbidity and mortality through the ages. With the advent of HIV there has recently been a resurgence of syphilis. The stages and symptoms of syphilis have been discussed elsewhere.
61	N	Urea and electrolytes ➢ Cisplatin is nephrotoxic and ototoxic. Urea and electrolytes and ideally serial pure tone audiograms are used to monitor toxicity. ➢ Cisplatin is a platinum based chemotherapy agent commonly used in head and neck cancer. It acts by inducing chloride cross linking between

		DNA bases. This interferes with mitosis and induces apoptosis. ➢ Nephrotoxicity is a dose related oxygen free radical based side effect that can be prevented by adequate fluid hydration and monitoring of creatinine clearance. ➢ Ototoxicity is caused by oxygen free radicals created by cisplatin or its ability to bind to melanin in the stria vascularis. Ototoxicity is irreversible and made more likely if cisplatin is given with aminoglycoside antibiotics.
62	G	Liver function test ➢ Sodium valproate is hepatotoxic and hence liver function monitoring is necessary. ➢ Valproic acid blocks voltage gated sodium channels and hence its use in epilepsy. It also promotes the neurotransmission of GABA and has thus been used for bipolar disease and major depression. ➢ The most severe side effect of this medication is fulminant hepatic failure and occurs when a patient first starts taking the medication. ➢ This class of medication has been successfully used in ENT to help treat facial neuralgias. The most commonly

		used is amitriptyline and gabapentin. Doses must be titrated up and so treatment can take many weeks. Patients are told to increase the medication at regular intervals until either the pain is well controlled or the side effects are unbearable.
63	L	Serum and urine osmolality ➢ This patient has developed diabetes insipidus (DI). This is a condition characterized by excessive thirst and excretion of large amounts of severely diluted urine. There are two main types of DI. The most common type in humans is central DI, caused by a deficiency of arginine vasopressin (AVP), also known as antidiuretic hormone. The second common type of DI is nephrogenic diabetes insipidus, which is caused by an insensitivity of the kidneys to ADH. It can also be an iatrogenic artifact of drug use. ➢ The condition can occur after head injury, meningitis, sepsis, or occasionally post operatively. It is in essence a failure of the kidney to concentrate urine. This leads to high volume fluid loss. The plasma becomes concentrated and this is reflected by a hypernatraemia and hyperosmolality.

		Since the kidney cannot concentrate urine well without ADH the urine sodium will be low and osmolalty also low. ➢ Diagnosis is made by water deprivation test. When the pateint is not allowed water, the kidney should be able to concentrate urine and reduce diuresis. If this does not occur than DI can be diagnosed. Next nasal desmopressin is given if the situation is reversed than it can be assumed that the pituitary was not secreting enough ADH (intracranial DI). If it doesn't reverse the situation nephrogenic DI is diagnosed. ➢ Treatment is meticulous sodium and fluid balance for disease that is only expected to last for a few days. If disease is protracted than desmopressin can be given for central DI and thiazide diuretics for nephrogenic DI.
64	K	RAST ➢ This test is suitable for patients who are unable to have a skin prick test, but is not as sensitive for air borne allergens. It has high reproducibility and specificity. It can be used in patients with severe eczema and on antihistamines, both of which preclude

		the use of skin prick testing. It can also be used when adding the allergen onto the patient has a high risk of anaphylaxis. ➢ This investigation works on the premise that allergic reactions are IgE mediated. Blood samples are taken and serum is separated from blood. The allergen is bound to an insoluble material and the patient's serum is added. If the patient has an allergic reaction to the added mixture. The antibody specifically binds to IgE. If IgE has remained bound to the allergen then the radiolabeled antibody will attach to it and light up. This indicates allergy to that substrate. This is carried out for numerous suspected allergens. ➢ A patient who has reducing allergy may still have IgE to the substrate and thus be shown to be allergic.
65	A	ACE ➢ This patient has signs and symptoms consistent with sarcoidosis. Angiotensin converting enzyme (ACE) catalyses the conversion of angiotensin I to angiotensin II in both the pulmonary and renal endothelial cells. It is raised in sarcoidosis and probably due to activated macrophages.

		➢ 25% of patients have lupus pernio and <6% have parotitis. Peripheral lymphadenopathy is seen 30%. Acute sarcoid is more common in caucasians and is more likely to completely resolve over two years. ➢ Staging of the disease depends on pulmonary findings and forms the basis of treatment. Stage I is bilateral hilar lymphadenopathy and Stage II is bilateral hilar lymphadenopathy with parenchymal infiltrates. Stage III is interestingly parenchymal infiltrates without hilar lymphadenopathy and Stage IV involves fibrosis. Stage I treatment does not require treatment. ➢ Diagnosis is clinical but helped by radiology and histology. Blood tests for ACE and calcium are often used for corroboration. ➢ Treatment is steroids and surgery for disease that has caused mass effect.
66	M	Streptococcus pneumonia ➢ Streptococcus pneumoniae is a normal inhabitant of the upper respiratory tract and this is due to its ability to adhere and replicate. It can progress from here to nasopharynx, sinuses and Eustachian tube etc. ➢ Infections are prevented by the normal

		mucociliary clearance. If this is affected infections can ensue. Activation of complement and release of weak toxin pneumolysin (which causes release of TNF alpha) are implicated in the clinical severity of the disease. ➢ It is the leading causes of bacterial infection in children and the elderly. It is a common pathogen that is responsible for many upper respiratory tract and ENT infections. (e.g. sinusitis, otitis media, pneumonia). ➢ Streptococcus pneumoniae is a lancet-shaped gram positive cocci. They are immotile and do not form spores. It is a fermentative aerotolerant anaerobe and needs to be cultured on blood agar, as blood contains the catalase necessary to reduced hydrogen peroxide produced by the bacteria. It forms in 2's or in chains. ➢ It is treated with penicillin based antibiotics.
67	J	Pseudomonas aeruginosa ➢ Pseudomonas aeruginosa is a gram negative bacterium found in soil and ground water. Half of all Pseudomonas species produce the blue green pigment called pyocyanin. It is a motile bacterium with a single polar flagellum.

		It is one of the fastest moving unicellular organisms in pond water. ➢ In nature it is often found in a biofilm attached to a substance. Pseudomonas has a predilection for moist environments. Its optimum growth temperature is 37°C but it can withstand heat up to 42°C. It is resistant to a high concentration of salt and dyes. It does not require organic growth factors and it can use more than seventy five organic compounds for growth. ➢ Pseudomonas only becomes pathological when the host defenses are depleted. It is an opportunistic bacterium that secretes an extracellular protease which helps adherence and invasion. It forms biofilms easily which makes it difficult to treat. It is the most common cause of perichondritis and is implicated in chronic ear infections as well as necrotising otitis externa. ➢ Treatment is with quinolones.
68	K	Staphylococcus aureus ➢ Staphylococcus aureus is an aerobic gram positive coccal bacterium. It is a nonmotile facultative anaerobe. ➢ Staphylococcus causes a wide variety

		of suppurative infections such as boils, styes and furunculosis. It also causes more serious infections such as pneumonia, mastitis, meningitis and urinary tract infections. It can also cause deep seated infections like osteomyelitis and endocarditis. ➢ Staph aureus is a major cause of nosocomial infections. It can cause food poisoning by release of enterotoxins and toxic shock syndrome through release of superantigens. Staph aureus quickly colonizes foreign material such as sutures and can be therefore difficult to treat. It requires a break in the skin for infection to start, via hair follicles, cuts or indwelling lines. It is often a cause of the superimposed bacterial pneumonias after a viral infection. ➢ Staphyloccocus aureus shows resistance for antiseptics and disinfectants, like quaternary ammonium compounds and this may explain why it survives so well in a hospital environment.
69	G	Klebsiella ➢ Atrophic rhinosinusitis results from destruction of the normal respiratory epithelium and transition to a

<table>
<tr><td></td><td></td><td>noncilated squamous epithelium, loss of mucociliary clearance and accumulation of stagnant mucous. This milieu facilitates acute and chronic infection (wet phase), and eventual sclerosis with epistaxis and chronic bloody crusts (dry phase).
<ul>
<li>Atrophic rhinitis is commonly associated with Klebsiella which has also become important pathogens in nosocomial infections. Klebsiella is a gram negative, lactose fermenting, non-motile, aerobic rod shaped bacterium with a prominent polysaccharide capsule.</li>
<li>The main determinant of its pathogenicity is its capsule which prevents against phagocytosis. It also protects bacteriocidal sera factors. This is done by inhibiting uptake of complement C3b. Lipopolysaccharide on the capsule prevent assembly of a membrane attack complex.</li>
<li>Rhinoscleroma is caused by Klebsiella and results in a reduction in local immunity. Treatment includes long term antibiotics.</li>
</ul></td></tr>
<tr><td>70</td><td>F</td><td>Haemophilus influenzae
<ul>
<li>This child has epiglottis and the history of no vaccination is significant.</li>
</ul></td></tr>
</table>

		Haemophilus influenzae is a non-motile gram negative rod-shaped bacterium. H. influenzae can cause serious invasive disease especially in young children. The most virulent strain is H. influenzae type b (Hib), which accounts for more than 95% of H. influenzae infections in children and half of infections in adults. This is protected against with the Hib vaccine. ➢ Hib may cause bacteraemia, meningitis epiglottitis etc. Non-encapsulated and non-typeable, H. influenzae strains cause mucosal infections, including exacerbations of chronic bronchitis and otitis media. ➢ Gram stain turns up pink if the bacterium is negative. If the bacterium is cocci shaped then it is Neisseria, coccoid shaped rods are Haemophilus or pertussis. If the bacterium is rod shaped it is placed onto a lactose agar. Lactose fermenters are Klebsiella and E coli. Lactose non fermenters are either oxidase positive (Pseudomonas) or negative (Salmonella).
71	C	Haemophilia A ➢ A common X-linked coagulation disorder with an incidence of 1:10,000 males. It is one of the first described

		genetic disorders and occurs due to a deficiency in clotting factor 8. ➢ Haemophilia A makes up 80% of haemophilias. Activated factor 8 is needed to convert factor 10 into activated factor 10. Its use is predominantly on the intrinsic pathway. This causes a high tendency to spontaneous bleeding. The gene for factor 8 is located on the long arm of the X chromosome. ➢ The majority of mutations on this gene (45%) are inversion type. Haemophilia A is the most common X linked disease and the second most common factor deficiency after von Willebrand disease. ➢ Although the disease is X linked it can be present in girls. This can be due to lyonisation of the normal X chromosome gene, Turner's syndrome (XO genotype), or both X chromosomes being affected (maternal carrier and paternal sufferer). ➢ A high proportion of these patients who were given blood product transfusions before 1985 were infected with HIV, with AIDS accounting for 55% of all haemophilia deaths in the 1990's. These infections are only historically

<table>
<tr><td></td><td></td><td><ul><li>important as screening techniques have improved so much.</li><li>Patients are given intermittent factor 8 to prevent joint damage. This dose will have to be increased before surgery. This is best done in conjunction with a haematologist.</li></ul></td></tr>
<tr><td>72</td><td>I</td><td>Thalassemia trait<ul><li>This disorder has numerous defects of gene for either alpha- or beta-globulin chain of haemoglobin, leading to imbalance to relative amounts of the chains. In endemic areas of malaria, it is the most common single-gene disease as it offers some protection.</li><li>Many disorders may be due wholly or partly to genetic factors which can be divided into three main groups:<ul><li>Single gene disorders (e.g. CF, Haemophilia A, NF, Osteogenesis imperfecta)</li><li>Chromosomal disorders (e.g. Down trisomy 18 and 13, turner and Prader Willi)</li><li>Multifactorial disorders (cleft lip and palate, congenital heart disease, neural tube defect)</li></ul></li><li>Single-gene defects are due to mutant genes and it may be present on one</li></ul></td></tr>
</table>

			chromosome or on both. In either case, the cause is a specific critical error in the genetic information. Mitochondrial transmitted diseases may be considered a special type of single-gene disorder. ➢ In chromosome disorders, the defect is due to an excess or deficiency of the genes contained in the whole chromosome or segments of the chromosome. The celebrated example is an extra copy of chromosome 21 which leads to Down's syndrome, even though no individual gene on the chromosome is abnormal. Collectively chromosomal disorders are fairly common, affecting 7 of 1000 live born infants and accounts for approximately half of all spontaneous first-trimester abortions. ➢ Multifactorial disorders are responsible for a number of developmental conditions resulting in congenital malformations. There is no single defect in the genetic information but rather a collection of small variations, which together may produce or predispose to a problem. Multi-factorial conditions tend to run in families and may involve

		environmental factors.
73	B	T1 N1 ➢ An important prognostic predictor for oral cancer is the clinicopathologic stage which describes the cancer developmental phase, and is established according to several criteria: (1) the tumor size, (2) the cancer location, and (3) the cancer extent (how far it has spread). ➢ The most common staging system used for oral cancer is the American Joint Committee on Cancer (AJCC) TNM system. The TNM system refers to:(T) the tumor features -size and invasion level; (N) the lymph nodes involved—lymph nodes are part of the body immune system; (M) the cancer metastasis—metastasis stage is the last developmental cancer stage when the cancer has spread to distal organs (organs situated far from the origin point).
74	G	T2N2a
75	J	T2N3
76	F	Non-disjunction ➢ This is the commonest mechanism involved in trisomy 21. Down's syndrome may also be caused by

		Robertsonian translocation which occurs between two acrocentric chromosomes by fusion at or near the centromere, with the loss of the short arms. ➢ A mild form of Down may be due to mosaicism in which there are two or more cell lines, derived from a single zygote but differing genetically because of post-zygotic mutation. ➢ Please refer to Paper 4 for full understanding of pathophysiology of Down syndrome.
77	M	Tumour suppressor gene ➢ Unicellular organisms are highly efficient at relentless propagation. Mutations in their genes do not normally preclude replication. In fact this may confer an environmental advantage to them which they can pass onto their next generation. ➢ However, in multicellular organisms, if a cell in a tissue undergoes a spontaneous mutation and passes on the gene it could prove catastrophic for the tissue/organ. There are genes programmed into our genome that represent multiple tumour suppressor genes. These genes are activated when the cell is behaving without the

		interest of the overall tissue. They code for proteins that eventually lead to apoptosis, or programmed cell death. However, if these abort pathways are dysfunctional then a cell that is behaving without the overall tissue's interests (as in cancer) can be allowed to grow and multiply. ➢ Luckily we have two copies of each gene and when one tumour suppressor gene is no longer working the other one can take over. This leads to the two hit hypotheses of tumour suppressor genes. It is likely in a pre-cancer state a person has an inherent defect in one copy of a tumour suppressor gene. The patient lives for many years without noting any problems. However, at some stage due to environmental stresses the second, and only functional, copy of the tumour suppressor gene undergoes mutation and stops working. Now this cell line is primed for tumour. ➢ P53 is the most widely implicated tumour suppressor gene in human cancer and it resides on chromosome 17. Mutations on this gene are recessive for the reason we discussed above. Oncogenes however exert a

		dominant effect and mutat on in just one copy of these genes ca1 lead to uncontrolled cell replication.
78	A	Allele ➢ Genes come in pairs, with one copy inherited from each parent. Many genes come in a number of variant forms, known as alleles. A dominant allele prevails over a normal allele. A recessive gene only becomes phenotypically apparent if its counterpart allele on the other chromosome becomes inactivated or lost. ➢ A simple example of this can be seen in cystic fibrosis. The allele for this disease is recessive. If a patient has one copy of this dysfunctional gene than its counterpart allele will prevail and the patient will have a normal phenotype. However, if both alleles are affected by the diseased gene than the patient will suffer from cystic fibrosis. ➢ In a second example of Huntington's disease the condition is inherited in a dominant fashion. This means that if one allele is affectec the patient will have the disease. ➢ The chance of passing on a recessive gene to the next generation is 1 in 2. If

		both parents are carriers then the chance of the offspring having the disease (having both copies of the diseased allele) is 1 in 4, which remains the same for each offspring. The chance of passing on a dominant gene to the next generation is 1 in 2 (as long as the disease lets you live long enough to reproduce). The chance of the offspring having the disease is still 1 in 2 in these diseases. ➢ However, most diseases and traits don't follow simple patterns of inheritance. Firstly not all mutated alleles lead to disease. Even with mutation of the oncogene BRCA1 (breast cancer susceptibility) the risk of disease by the age of 65 is 80% not 100%. This quality of whether a mutated gene will produce phenotypic disease is known as penetrance.
79	C	Meiosis ➢ Meiosis is cell division for eukaryotic cells. It involves a single cell with 23 pairs of chromosomes becoming four cells with 23 chromosomes each. This haploid cell will either form a sperm or an egg, and during copulation when these two cells merge during fertilisation the fetus will have a 23

pairs of chromosomes (diploid).

- The steps are as follows: Prophase, metaphase, anaphase and telophase. There is a step Prophase I that is individual to meiosis. The normal prophase involves DNA replication and therefore 23 pairs of chromosomes become 46 pairs of chromosomes. The unique step involves the duplicated chromosomes lining up next their counterpart (e.g. maternally derived chromosome 17 lies next to paternally derived chromosome 17). This phase allows exchange of genes between chromosomes.
- An example would be a subject who has a gene for blue eyes on chromosome 17 from his mother and brown eyes from his father on his other chromosome 17. He can pass down either chromosome to his offspring, and they may have blue or brown eyes depending on who the subject mates with. However if this crossing over process has occurred at the locus where eye colour is coded on chromosome 17, the subject may transmit only his father's chromosome 17 but this may have the gene for blue eyes derived from his mother's

		chromosome 17. This process allows for far greater genetic heterogeneity than simple mitosis.
80	H	Phenotype ➢ This refers to the observed features of the individual and is dependent on the genotype and environment in which it is expressed. The genotype is the genetic constitution. The phenotypic expressive of a genotype is dependent on the heterogeneity of the alleles, the dominant-recessive interaction of the alleles and the penetrance of the allele. ➢ In the following example phenotypic variation is shown. A patient who has a defective gene for a dominantly inherited condition will still possess a normal gene. However, due to the dominant nature of inheritance on the gene, the normal gene is silenced and the abnormal gene expressed. However, some autosomal dominant conditions have poor penetrance, i.e. despite having a functioning copy of the mutated gene they will not necessarily have the disease. This is an example of how having the genotype does not necessarily mean you will express it as a phenotype.
81	H	Neural presbycusis

			➢ Presbycusis is the age related reduction in hearing and affects 50% of people above the age of 75. ➢ The underlying mechanism is thought to be the interplay of genetics and environmental factors. Reduced blood flow in the vasa nervorum in the internal acoustic meatus occurs with age. This reduction is thought to cause the release of oxygen free radicals which damage the mitochondrial DNA of the cochlea and therefore cause a reduction in oxidative phosphorylation. This in turn affects neural structures. Indeed reduced blood flow in the vasa nervorum has been shown to increase damage to mitochondrial DNA in the cochlea. There are six main types of presbycusis: sensory, neural, strial, cochlear conductive, intermediate and mixed. ➢ Neural presbycusis is caused by atrophy of the cochlea nerve cells and central nerve pathways. Audiometric findings include gradual hearing loss with a moderate slope toward the high frequencies and a disproportionately severe decrease in speech discrimination. This difficulty with speech discrimination makes hearing

		loss refractory to amplification in many cases. Atrophy of the spiral ganglion and nerves of the osseous spiral lamina occurs mainly in the basal turn of the cochlea. Corti's organ is largely intact, as opposed to the condition in sensory presbycusis.
82	J	Strial presbycusis. ➢ Strial presbycusis may be familial and progresses slowly. It affects the stria vascularis that is responsible for supporting the other cells of the cochlea. Therefore all frequencies tend to be affected. The hearing loss associated with strial presbycusis is a flat sensory loss that begins in the third through sixth decades and progresses slowly. Speech discrimination is generally good and no recruitment occurs. Patients do well with amplification. ➢ The characteristic pathologic findings are atrophy of the stria vascularis, which may be either patchy in the basal and apical turns or diffuse. Corti's organ and the spiral ganglion cells are usually unaffected. Studies have found high cholesterol levels correlate to higher incidence of presbycusis. The use of atorvastatin does not appear to

		be protective. ➢ Intermediate presbycusis is similar to strial but with poor speech discrimination.
83	E	Enlarged vestibular aqueduct syndrome ➢ The vestibular aqueduct is a tiny canal shielded by the temporal bone, one of the densest bones in the body. It houses the endolymphatic duct and sac. An enlarged vestibular aqueduct (EVA) can be associated with genetic conditions such as Pendred syndrome, which affects thyroid function and hearing, and branchiootorenal syndrome, which affects kidney function and hearing. ➢ It can also be associated with anatomical problems such as Mondini deformity, when the cochlea develops incompletely. ➢ When EVA causes hearing loss or balance symptoms, it is referred to as enlarged vestibular aqueduct syndrome (EVAS). Some people are born with hearing loss, but most hear normally in the first years of life and then notice losses later in childhood, or less commonly in adolescence or early adulthood. Often, this occurs after a minor or major head impact, upper

		respiratory infection or air pressure trauma.
84	I	Sensory presbycusis. ➢ Sensory presbycusis affects the hair cells of the organ of Corti and their supporting milieu. Hair cells at the basal turn are more affected than those at the apex. The end result is hearing loss at high frequencies. This loss is often higher than speech frequencies and so speech discrimination is unaffected until the disease progresses. ➢ The audiometric findings in sensory presbycusis include an abrupt high-frequency sensorineural loss with slow, symmetric progression, usually beginning in middle age. ➢ Pathologic lesions are limited to the first few millimetres of the basal turn of the cochlea. Flattening and atrophy of Corti's organ result from loss of hair cells and supporting cells. Lipofuscin, the aging pigment, also accumulates.
85	G	Inner ear conductive presbycusis. ➢ Both inner ear conductive presbycusis and atrophy of the spiral ligament cause bilateral symmetric sensorineural loss with an upward slope toward the high frequencies and

		preserved speech discrimination. ➢ The anatomic correlate to conductive sensorineural hearing loss is not completely understood, but it is hypothesized that the functional loss is due to stiffness of the basilar membrane, which correlates with its anatomic shape. ➢ The histopathologic pattern of atrophy of the spiral ligament includes different degrees of pathologic changes progressive throughout the patient's life. It is most noticeable in the apical turn and least in the basal turn. Cystic degeneration may cause detachment of Corti's organ from the lateral cochlear wall, resulting in hearing loss.
86	F	Type C2 ➢ Tympanometry applies a tone to the external auditory canal and measure its reflection back to a microphone. The pressure in the canal is varied to see at which pressure impedance is lowest and immitane highest. ➢ The tympanic membrane separates the outer ear from the middle ear. It vibrates in relation to sound. And the more compliant it is to the vibration of sound the more energy is transferred to the ossicles. Therefore the only

		factor that should affect how much the drum moves is the intensity and frequency of the sound. Pressure differences across the drum would impact on the ability of the drum to emit/impede sound energy. ➢ Therefore we have a Eustachian tube that equilibrates the environment behind the drum (middle ear) to that in front of it (external ear). When the Eustachian tube is blocked the respiratory epithelium of the middle ear absorbs the air and creates a vacuum. This causes the drum to be sucked into the middle ear. In so doing it is no longer able to emit/impede sound optimally and this leads to a conductive hearing loss. ➢ By varying the pressure in the external ear we are able to estimate the pressure in the middle ear. As when the two pressures are equal sound immittance will be greatest. In this case we see that the highest peak occurs in negative pressure range and therefore we can assume the pressure behind the drum is negative and the Eustachian tube is not correctly functioning.
87	B	Type Ad

		➢ Type A traces imply that the peak of the immittance curve is it atmospheric pressure and that there is no issue with pressure differentials (normal compliance is 0.3–1.6 mL/equivalent air volume). ➢ However, there are two anomalous types of Type A trace. Type As (stiff) refers to a small peak. This tells you that sound energy is not getting through as efficiently as expected. It is seen in tympanosclerosis and otosclerosis. If this is associated with a conductive hearing loss and a normal tympanic membrane, stapedial reflexes should be performed and stapedotomy should be considered. Type Ad (discontinuous) refers to a hypermobile drum and therefore the immittance of sound into the middle ear is high (as is the peak on the graph). This is seen after ossicular fractures or from a flaccid drum. If this is associated with a conductive hearing loss it should be first investigated with a CT scan and if this has not provided an answer tympanotomy may be necessary.
88	C	Type As ➢ Type As implies that the compliance or

		acoustic admittance of the tympanic membrane is low (or shallow) and this may occur in otosclerosis or severe tympanosclerosis. The normal compliance is 0.3–1.6 mL/equivalent air volume. The acoustic admittance is dominated by the stiffness of the tympanic membrane, particularly at low frequencies. At higher frequencies the most important factor in determining impedance is the mass of the ossicular chain. ➢ The following points regarding tympanic membrane perforation are worth noting: 1. Type B trace is flat and suggests one of two things: tympanic membrane perforation or fluid behind the drum. In the case of middle ear fluid, the pressure behind the drum is far greater than atmospheric; therefore there is a conductive block to sound immittance. The reason no peak is seen relate to the fact the tympanometry machine is unable to generate pressure high enough to equal that of the fluid behind the drum. To generate enough air jet pressure to match fluid

pressure behind the drum would cause damage to surrounding structures and is avoided. Therefore in these patients we are seeing the build up to the peak.

2. In patients who have a perforation it is impossible to get a peak as the drum is unable to make a standard wave that allows a peak in sound reflection. Since varying the pressure in the external auditory canal will instantly alter the pressure in the middle ear this has no effect on the curve.
3. However, these two conditions can be differentiated using the measure ear canal volume. If the drum is intact this will read the normal volume of around 1 cm^2. If there is a perforation it will read the volume in the external auditory canal and the middle ear and mastoid giving a larger reading. In reality these two conditions do not need to be differentiated by tympanometry as simple microscopic examination will yield the diagnosis.
4. If a perforation is seen, the conductive hearing loss is linearly

		related to the size of the perforation and not its location. If a large air bone gap is seen with only a small perforation, it indicates distal pathology. When planning a tympanoplasty for a perforation there is greater success if there has been no Eustachian tube dysfunction. The history of Eustachian tube dysfunction can be assessed by a CT of the temporal bone which demonstrates good pneumatisation of the mastoid if the Eustachian tube has done its job effectively through the years. Not all patients will require CT and this is where the ear canal volume may prove useful. A patient with a known perforation and only slight increase in external canal volume is likely to have a poorly ventilated middle ear. This should be anticipated addressed as part of management.
89	M	Titanium ➢ Grade I microtia shows a less than normal development of the pinna but full development of the external auditory canal. ➢ Grade II shows a partially developed

		pinna with a stenotic or collapsed external auditory canal. ➢ Grade III microtia, which is the most common type, has minimal pinna development, with absent ear canal and drum. ➢ Cochlear function is maintained and so the aim should be restore conduction to the cochlea and provide an aesthetically pleasing ear. Reconstruction of the ear using rib graft can be done at 7-years-old. This will continue to grow with the child. ➢ Hearing is normally restored using a bone anchored hearing aid. These are secured using titanium screws to the cranium. At the same sitting screws can be inserted for prosthesis. Prostheses are made of silicone and look very good. They can be removed easily and changed. However, they do not grow and are not appropriate for frequent changes as the child grows. Titanium is used as it osseointegrates into the skull bone and is safe to MRI in the future.
90	D	Gutta Percha ➢ Gutta Percha is a tropical tree found in the Malaysian peninsula. Its sap, also called Gutta Percha, has been used for

		nearly 200 years and is inelastic latex. It was originally used to insulate underwater cables as it has great insulator properties and bio-inertness. ➤ It has been used in dentistry for around 80 years during root canal surgery to obliterate the root cavity hole. ➤ Following maxillectomy for cancer the cavity can either be reconstructed or obturated depending on surgeon/patient choice and the availability of a restorative dentist. ➤ This can prevent aspiration of food into the nasal cavity but also allow the soft tissues of the face to sit proud without sinking into the cavity.
91	E	Hydroxyapatite ➤ The purpose of a mastoidectomy it to improve drainage of the mastoid air cells into the antrum and middle ear. It is also the purpose of the procedure to remove the underlying disease. The end result should be a dry ear. However on occasion this does not occur and a solution has to be found. ➤ The main causes for persistently discharging ear after mastoidectomy include incomplete removal of disease (residing in unopen air cells, facial recess or sinus tympani), high facial

		ridge (which prevents easy migration of squamous debris from the cavity into the external auditory canal—the facial ridge is the posterior canal Wall remnant), inadequate canal meatoplasty, and too large a cavity. ➢ The first step is to perform a detailed examination to ensure there is no recurrence or residual disease, a high facial ridge or a narrow canal. Regular aural toilet should next be done to try and keep the cavity infection free. A CT scan should be performed to examine for unopened cells that harbour disease. If all the above is done and there is no resolution then a mastoid obiteration should be planned. This can be done using hydroxyapatite, which act as a substrate for osteoneogenesis.
92	L	Teflon ➢ In otosclerosis the disease affects the stapes foot plate which becomes fixed to the oval window. Surgical cure involves bypassing the sclerotic bone. This is done by drilling a hole in the stapes foot plate. A piston is placed through the hole and connected directly to the incus. Thus movement of the incus will cause movement of the piston and eventually the oval

		window. ➢ The material used in type of stapes prostheses commonly used in this country is Teflon - Polytetrafluoroethylene – based. The top part on the prosthesis must be stretched so that it can fit around the long process of the incus. As a result of the intrinsic memory it contracts and fix snugly around the ossicle. ➢ Other types of prosthesis (like the SMart piston) are made of nitinol and fluoroplastic. They hook can be heated and caused to rapidly contract around the long process of the incus. This makes placement easier, especially if laser heat is used. There have been few instances of overly tight application of the prosthesis around the incus which leads to necrosis. Inadequate fitting may result in the prosthesis falling off.
93	H	Platinum ➢ A cochlear implant is made of many parts. Sound is received by a microphone and then filtered to asses show the electrodes should be activated. The processor works on a complex series of Fast Fourier transformations that splits sound into constituent parts, and prioritizes

		speech frequencies (each vowel has a fundamental frequency. ➢ These algorithms try to recognise the vowel and then emphasise its features. These strategies emphasise the transmission of spectral aspects of speech. The processed sound is then transmitted (via a transmitter) via radiowaves. This equipment is placed over skin. There are no wires going between transmitter and receiver, as signals pass via radiowaves. The receive sits beneath skin but is magnetically attached to the transmitter through a magnet. The receiver translates the processed sound information and controls the electric current to the electrode. The electrode array is made from rubber silicone while the electrodes are platinum or a similar highly conductive material. They insert into the round window and selectively activate different parts of the cochlear nerve.
94	K	Visual reinforcement audiometry ➢ Some children do not accept that a headphone is put on their head or insert earphones are inserted in their ear. For some children, the only way to conduct an audiometric evaluation is

to present sounds by means of loudspeakers. In order to achieve correct results the test environment must be calibrated prior to the actual test. In order for the child to respond to an audible sound, it is linked to visual signals like funny, colourful pictures. The procedure is called Visual Reinforcement Audiometry.

- Every time after a sound is presented a picture follows some seconds later. After a couple of times the child realizes a pattern that there is a picture after the sound. Actually the child is not interested in the sound but in the picture. An audible sound makes the child looking for the picture. Therefore, every search reaction following a sound suggests that the previous sound was audible.
- For hearing instrument benefit evaluation, Visual Reinforcement Audiometry is done twice: first without and then with hearing instrument. The difference between these two results is the improvement provided by the hearing instrument. Visual Reinforcement Audiometry is one part of a whole test battery for children, which also includes Tympanometry,

		Otoacoustic Emissions and Auditory Brainstem Response.

95	A	Auditory brainstem response
		➢ The auditory brainstem response (ABR) is an auditory evoked potential extracted from ongoing electrical activity in the brain and recorded via electrodes placed on the scalp. It is commonly carried out under a general anaesthesia. The resulting recording is a series of vertex positive waves of which I through V are evaluated.
		➢ These waves, labeled with roman numerals, occur in the first 10 msec after onset of an auditory stimulus and are easily remember using the mnemonic ECOLI:
		    ➢ **E** – generated by the peripheral portion of the Eight cranial nerve
		    ➢ C– generated by the cochlear nucleuscertral portion of cranial nerve VIII
		    ➢ O– generated by the Olivary complex cochlear nucleus
		    ➢ L– generated by the Lateral lemniscus
		    ➢ **I** – generated by the Inferior colliculus
		➢ The ABR is considered an exogenous

		response because it is dependent upon external factors.
96	F	Pure tone audiometry ➢ Pure tone audiometry (PTA) is the cornerstone hearing test used to identify hearing threshold levels of an individual. It enables determination of the degree, type and configuration of a hearing loss and therefore provides the basis for diagnosis and management. ➢ PTA is a subjective, behavioral measurement of hearing threshold, as it relies on patient response to pure tone stimuli. Therefore, PTA is used on adults and children old enough to cooperate with the test procedure. ➢ As with most clinical tests, calibration of the test environment, the equipment and the stimuli to ISO standards is needed before testing proceeds. PTA only measures thresholds, rather than other aspects of hearing such as sound localisation. ➢ However, there are benefits of using PTA over other forms of hearing test, such as click auditory brainstem response. PTA provides ear specific thresholds, and uses frequency specific pure tones to give place specific

		responses, so that the configuration of a hearing loss can be identif ed (Figures 3.48a and 3.48b). As PTA uses both air and bone conduction audiometry, the type of loss can also be identified via the air-bone gap.
97	E	Otoacoustic emissions ➢ Otoacoustic emissions (OAEs) are intrinsic sounds produced from outer hair cells and are considered to be related to the amplification function of the cochlea. ➢ OAEs are currently evoked using three different methodologies. Stimulus frequency OAEs (SFOAEs) are measured during the application of a pure-tone stimulus, and are detected by the vectorial difference between the stimulus waveform and the recorded waveform (which consists of the sum of the stimulus and the OAE). Transient-evoked OAEs (TEOAEs or TrOAEs) are evoked using a click (broad frequency range) or tone burst (brief duration pure tone) stimulus. The evoked response from a click covers the frequency range up to around 4 k Hz, while a toneburst will elicit a response from the region that has the same frequency as the pure tone.

		➢ Otoacoustic emissions are clinically important because they are the basis of a simple, non-invasive, test for hearing defects in newborn babies and in children who are too young to cooperate in conventional hearing tests. ➢ Otoacoustic emissions are fundamental to the national programmes for the universal hearing screening of newborn babies. Periodic early childhood hearing screenings program are also utilising OAE technology. OAE screening and follow-up practices in those early childhood educational settings. ➢ The primary screening tool is a test for the presence of a click-evoked OAE. Otoacoustic emissions also assist in differential diagnosis of cochlear and higher level hearing losses. ➢ Three basic steps to interpretation of a OAE involve assessing the stimulus, probe stability and response or signal to noise ratio (remember SPR).
98	M	Two-way analysis of variance (ANOVA) ➢ Analysis of variance is a statistical tool to assess whether the means of several groups are equal or not. In its simplest

		form it is the equivalent of a t-test for multiple groups. ➢ Multiple t-tests could be done for the same study however this would increase your chance of a type I error. ➢ In this study we are assessing the effect of thyroidectomy on calcium levels but also the effect of the grade of surgeon. ➢ The three null hypotheses are that 1. Thyroidectomy has no effect on the calcium levels, 2. Grade of the surgeon has no effect on calcium levels 3. There is no interaction between the grade of the surgeon and the type of thyroidectomy. ➢ There are three outcome measures (3 point calcium results – interval parametric data) and two possible affecting variables (whether surgery affects results and grade of surgeon – senior/junior) ➢ An ANOVA should used to analyze all the results. But since there are two variables a two way ANOVA should be used.
99	I	One-way Analysis of variance (ANOVA) ➢ When deciding on a statistical test the following considerations should be made: The type and number of

		outcomes measures (this is parametric interval data), the use of central measure (mean), the number of variables (4). ➢ For this case an ANOVA is best used. In this group the data is parametric and expected to be distributed normally; therefore we should investigate parametric tests. ➢ The next question is how many samples are there? In this case there are four. ➢ When there are more than two an ANOVA should be used. ➢ If there are two or less samples than a t-test should be considered. ➢ When there are more two samples and they are matched then a repeat measures ANOVA can be used. ➢ If however, they are not matched as in this case one has to consider independent variables. ➢ If there is only one than a one-way ANOVA is used and if there are two independent variables then a two-factor ANOVA is used.
100	F	Mann–Whitney U test ➢ Here again you have two groups or samples (from north and south) but only one variable (exam scores). The

data are parametric, ratio data that should be normally distributed. This means the scores are given on a scale (1–100%) and you would expect there to be a mean that is not dissimilar from the median, with a few students who score very highly and some who score very poorly.

- The next question is how many separate samples are there and in this case there are two samples and so a t-test should be used.
- The final question is whether the data are matched and in this case they are not so an independent measures t-test should be undertaken. If the data is thought not to be normally distributed from previous calculations than non parametric tests should be considered.
- Again there are two variables (North and South), so the options include Wilcoxon Chi squared and Mann–Whitney U test. Since the samples are not matched then Wilcoxon cannot be used. Since the scores can be ranked in order Mann–Whitney U test is appropriate otherwise Chi squared could have been used.

CHAPTER 4

Paper 4

EMI Questions (Q1-Q100)

For each stem, select one correct answer option.

Theme: Paediatric syndromes

Options for Questions 1–5:

A Alport syndrome
B Apert syndrome
C CHARGE syndrome
D Cogan's syndrome
E Crouzon syndrome
F Down's syndrome
G Goldenhar syndrome
H Pendred's syndrome
I Pierre–Robin sequence
J Refsum syndrome
K Treacher–Collins syndrome
L Usher's syndrome

For each of the following cases, select the single most likely syndrome. Each option may be used once, more than once or not at all.

1. A newborn boy presents with a cardiac murmur, ear abnormalities and choanal atresia.

2. A 2-year-old girl presents with deafness and retinitis pigmentosa.

3. A newborn girl presents with unilateral facial asymmetry and scoliosis.

4. A 3-year-old girl presents with bilateral conductive hearing loss, hypoplastic maxilla and syndactyl of the hands and feet.

5. A 7-year-old boy presents with upslanting palpebral fissure.

Theme: Facial nerve palsy

Options for Questions 6–10:

A Guillain Barre syndrome
B Heerfordt's syndrome
C Leprosy
D Lyme disease
E Maffucci syndrome
F Melkersson–Rosenthal syndrome
G Moebius syndrome
H Multiple sclerosis
I Myasthenia gravis
J Parotid tumour
K Syphilis
L Squamous cell carcinoma

For each of the following cases, select the single most likely diagnosis. Each option may be used once, more than once or not at all.

6. A 6-month-old boy presents with poor suckling reflex. On examination, he was noted to have bilateral squints and facial nerve palsies, which were present since birth. He was born at 40-weeks gestation by forceps delivery.
7. A 27-year-old man presents with intermittent facial nerve palsy and a swollen fissured tongue.
8. A 70-year old man presents with sabre-shaped tibia and unilateral facial nerve palsy.
9. A 22-year old male presents with deteriorating vision and unilateral facial nerve palsy.
10. A 47-year-old woman presents with fever, red eyes, unilateral facial nerve palsy and bilateral enlargements of the parotid glands.

Theme: Complications of otitis media

Options for 11–13:

A Bezold's abscess
B Citelli's abscess
C Extradural abscess
D Facial nerve palsy
E Hearing loss
F Labyrinthitis
G Lateral sinus thrombosis
H Meningitis
I Perforation of tympanic membrane
J Subdural abscess
K Subperiosteal abscess

L Tympanosclerosis

For each of the following cases, select the single most likely diagnosis. Each option may be used once, more than once or not at all.

11. A 45-year-old man presents with acute onset of nausea and vertigo. He is just recovering from a head cold. Examination reveals nystagmus, with the fast phase beating to the left.

12. A 3-year-old girl presents with painful left sided swelling in level 2 of the neck associated with otalgia. Ultrasound sound scan reveals the presence of a collection in the left digastric fossa.

13. A 63-year-old woman presents with fever, drowsiness, lethargy and facial weakness She has a history of cholesteatoma associated with foul smelling discharge.

Theme: Neck pathology

Options for Questions 14–18:

A Branchial cyst
B Cervical rib
C Cystic hygroma
D Glomus jugular tumour
E Goitre
F Laryngomalacia
G Metastatic carcinoma
H Pharyngeal pouch
I Sternomastoid tumour

J Subclavian artery aneurysm
K Thyroglossal cyst
L Tonsillar tumour
M Tonsillitis

For each of the following cases, select the single most likely diagnosis. Each option may be used once, more than once or not at all.

14. A 32-year-old pregnant woman presents with a uniformly enlarged thyroid.

15. A 26-year-old woman presents with a hard mass attached to C7.

16. A 28-year-old man presents with a pulsatile swelling in the lower aspect of the neck at the base of sternocleidomastoid. He experiences a cold hand on the same side.

17. A 50-year-old man presents with a 5–10 cm indistinct mass behind sternocleidomastoid muscle, below the thyroid cartilage. The lump is soft, smooth and compressible on palpation. He is just recovering from a chest infection.

18. A 50-year-old man present with a painless swelling in the upper lateral part of his neck on the left side, deep to and protruding from the anterior upper 1/3 of sternocleidomastoid muscle. It measured 5 cm in diameter and was smooth, non-tender and fluctuant.

Theme: Conditions of the voice

Options for Questions 19–22:

A Acute laryngitis
B Essential tremor
C Reinke's oedema
D Singer's nodules
E Singers nodules
F Spasmodic dysphonia
G Sulcus vocalis
H Vocal Cord granuloma
I Vocal cord palsy
J Vocal cord polyp

For each of the following cases, select the single most likely diagnosis. Each option may be used once, more than once or not at all.

19. A 36-year-old man presents with a hoarse voice, difficulty being heard, and is often confused for a woman on the telephone. Videostroboscopy shows a linear depression in the free edge of the true vocal cord.

20. A 45-year-old male patient presents with a foreign body sensation in throat, and intermittent voice break. Nasoendoscopy shows a unilateral midline mass arising from left vocal cord

21. A 56-year-old male smoker presents with hoarse and weak voice, and gets winded when trying to speak long sentences.

22. A 36-year-old female presents with an intermittent strained, strangled breaks in her voice. Her symptoms do not appear during laughing or singing.

Theme: Middle ear anatomy

Options for 23–27:

A Facial recess
B Internal auditory canal
C Petrotympanic fissure
D Processus cochleariformis
E Prussak's space
F Pyramidal eminence
G Scutum
H Sinus Tympani
I Stapedius
J Stylomastoid foramen
K Tensor Tympani

For each of the following anatomical statements, select the single most likely anatomical structure. Each option may be used once, more than once or not at all.

23. Exit route for chorda tympani from middle ear.

24. Innervated by the mandibular nerve.

25. Stapedius tendon exits from this structure to attach to stapes.

26. The lateral limit of the epitympanum.

27. The area between round window niche and the pyramidal eminence.

Theme: Salivary gland pathology

Options for Questions 28–30:

A	Acute sialadenitis
B	Mucoepidermoid Carcinoma
C	Mucous retention cyst
D	Mikulicz's Syndrome
E	Oncocytoma
F	Pleomorphic adenoma
G	Ranula
H	Sialolithiasis
I	Warthin's tumour

For each of the following cases, select the single most likely diagnosis. Each option may be used once, more than once or not at all.

28. A 34-year-old man presents with gradual facial swelling in the region of the ramus of the mandible and eyes. He complains of a dry mouth. He was recently diagnosis with sarcoidosis.

29. A 70-year-old man presents with a soft mass in the tail of his parotid on the left. He is a smoker. FNA shows papillary formations, cystic spaces and a supporting stroma of dense lymphoid tissue with follicles.

30. A 46-year-old woman presents with a blue, translucent swelling in the floor of her mouth.

Theme: Conditions of the pinna

Options for Questions 31–35:

A Auricular endochondral pseudocyst
B Basal cell carcinoma
C Chondrodermatitis nodularis helicis
D Gouty tophi
E Keratoacanthoma
F Pinna cellulitis
G Relapsing polychondritis
H Sebaceous cyst
I Squamous cell carcinoma
J Telephone ear

For each of the following cases, select the single most likely diagnosis. Each option may be used once, more than once or not at all.

31. A 65-year-old male farmer presents with a bleeding lesion on the upper part of the pinna. Examination reveals a 1 cm ulcerative lesion, with heaped up edges and a palpable level 2 lymph node.

32. A 56-year-old man presents with 8 mm mass on helix of right ear. The lesion is painful and tender to touch. He sleeps on his right, and now finds it uncomfortable. It is a well defined raised lesion with crusting. The crusting is removed to reveal a channel. At the periphery, intact epidermis is edematous and acanthotic. The dermis below the ulceration demonstrates homogeneous acellular collagen degeneration, with fibrin deposition.

33. A 45-year-old Caucasian female presents with a sudden onset of unilateral otalgia and erythema over right pinna. Has occurred once before, but was self resolving within 2 weeks. The patient reports they may have had trauma, but cannot be certain. On examination, there was swelling of the entire pinna, sparing the lobule. Histology shows infiltration of T lymphocytes,

34. An 18-year-old girl presents with a mass, which appeared on the lobule of her left ear. It is mobile under the skin. It recently became red and tender.

35. A 36-year-old Chinese male presents with a painless, fluctuant out-pouching of the upper anterior surface of the pinna. He admits he has had multiple minor traumatic insults to this site over the last 3 years. Histology shows dilated lymphatic system within normal tissue planes.

Theme: Audiological investigations

Options for Questions 36–39:

A Acoustic Reflex
B Auditory Brainstem Response
C Auditory response cradle
D Conditioned response audiometry
E Cortical evoked response audiometry
F Distraction testing
G Electrocochleography
H Free field testing
I Pure tone audiogram

J Stenger's test
K Tympanometry

For each of the following cases, select the single most appropriate diagnostic test. Each option may be used once, more than once or not at all.

36. A 39-year-old patient presents with suspected non-organic hearing loss.
37. A 3-month-old boy presents with possible congenital hearing loss.
38. An 8-month-old girl presents with suspicion of hearing loss
39. A 28-year-old woman presents with a GP diagnosis of otosclerosis, based on a Carhart notch on her pure tone audiogram and a type As tympanogram.

Theme: Figures pertaining to UK Guidelines in ENT practice for tonsillectomy

Options for Questions 40–41:

A 1 episode
B 2 episodes
C 3 episodes
D 4 episodes
E 5 episodes
F 6 episodes
G 7 episodes
H 8 episodes
I 9 episodes

J 10 episodes

For each of the following cases, select the single most appropriate selection criteria to consider for surgery. Each option may be used once, more than once or not at all.

40. The number of episodes/year of tonsillitis required for listing a patient for bilateral tonsillectomies.

41. The number of episodes of quinces required for listing a patient for bilateral tonsillectomies.

Theme: Eponymous names relevant to otolaryngology

Options for Questions 42–46:

A Haller cells

B Kuhn cells

C Kupffer cells

D Langerhans cells

E Langhan's cells

F Michaels's bodies

G Mikulicz's cells

H Onodi cells

I Reed–Sternberg cells

J Russell's bodies

K Schaumann's bodies

L Schwann cells

M Warthin–Finkeldey giant cells

For each of the following descriptions, select the single most likely corresponding eponymous name. Each option may be used once, more than once or not at all.

42. A multinucleated cell found in granulomatous conditions.

43. A neoplastic binucleated cell.

44. An air cell related to the maxillary sinus.

45. An air cell related to the sphenoid sinus.

46. Epithelial nest of cells thought to be the source of congenital cholesteatoma.

Theme: Thyroid pathology

Options for Questions 47–50:

A Anaplastic carcinoma
B De Quervain's thyroiditis
C Endemic goitre
D Follicular adenoma
E Follicular carcinoma
F Graves' disease
G Hashimoto's disease
H Lymphoma
I Medullary carcinoma
J Papillary carcinoma
K Riedel's thyroiditis

For each of the following cases, select the single most appropriate pathology. Each option may be used once, more than once or not at all.

47. A 65-year-old African man presents with a large, smooth goitre. He says it has been increasing in size for at least 15 years.

48. A 50-year-old woman presents with a painless, firm, neck swelling located on the right. Fine needle aspiration shows multiple compact follicles. Following a lobectomy, histology shows evidence of capsular and blood vessel invasion.

49. A 32-year-old woman presents with increasing weight gain, lethargy and neck swelling. On examination the patient has a firm rubbery goitre. Fine needle aspiration shows a diffuse lymphocytic/plasma cell infiltrate with the presence of lymphoid follicles and parenchymal atrophy.

50. A 40-year-old woman presents with a steadily enlarging lump at the base of the neck on the right. On examination there is a thyroid nodule, with associated lymphadenopathy. She has raised levels of calcitonin on TFTs.

Theme: House–Brackmann (HB) grading of facial nerve palsy

Options for Questions 51–53:

A HB Grade I
B HB Grade II
C HB Grade III
D HB Grade IV
E HB Grade V
F HB Grade VI

For each of the following cases, select the single most appropriate HB grade. Each option may be used once, more than once or not at all.

51. A 38-year-old man presents with normal symmetry and tone at rest, but no forehead movement and incomplete eye closure.

52. A 38-year-old man presents with normal symmetry, and tone at rest but moderate–good forehead movement and complete eye closure with effort. Close inspection reveals only slight facial weakness.

53. A 38-year-old man presents with no facial movements present.

Theme: Conditions of the ear canal

Options for Questions 54–58:

A	Canal stenosis or atresia
B	Ear canal polyp
C	Eczema
D	Exostoses
E	External auditory canal cholesteatoma
F	Foreign body
G	Furunculosis
H	Keratosis obturans
I	Necrotising otitis externa
J	Osteoma
K	Otitis externa
L	Pseudotympanic membrane
M	Pyogenic granuloma

N Squamous cell carcinoma of the external auditory canal

For each of the following cases, select the single most likely diagnosis. Each option may be used once, more than once or not at all.

54. A 25-year-old male surfer presents with recurrent otitis externa, and conductive hearing loss. Examination shows bilateral sessile masses adjacent to tympanic membrane in the external auditory canal.

55. A 35-year-old man presents with unilateral conductive hearing loss. Examination reveals a pedunculated mass extending from the bony cartilaginous junction of the external auditory canal.

56. A 69-year-old female presents with severe bilateral otalgia and conductive hearing loss. Otoscopy shows widened EAC medially, thickened tympanic membrane and hyperaemic skin with granulation tissue.

57. A 65-year-old female presents with chronic dull unilateral otalgia, otorrhoea and no hearing loss. Examination shows localised erosion posteroinferiorly in external auditory canal. Patient has had a myringoplasty 3 years ago.

58. A 57-year-old diabetic male presents with one month of unilateral purulent otorrhoea and severe otalgia. Examination shows granulation at bony-cartilaginous junction.

Theme: Skin lesions

Options for Questions 59–62:

A Acral lentiginous melanoma
B Basal cell carcinoma
C Benign naevus
D Keloid scar
E Keratoacanthoma
F Papilloma
G Sebaceous cyst
H Squamous cell carcinoma
I Superficial spreading malignant melanoma

For each of the following cases, select the single most likely diagnosis. Each option may be used once, more than once or not at all.

59. A 48-year-old man presents with an irregular lesion on the back of his neck, which has enlarged and started bleeding.

60. A 55-year-old male farmer presents with a lesion on his under the angle of the mandible, which grows rapidly and then regresses.

61. An 80-year-old man presents with a pearly edged lesion on the vertex of his scalp. He is a regular golfer.

62. A 48-year-old woman presents with an exophytic lesion in her nasal vestibule. It bleeds occasionally.

Theme: Ototoxic drugs

Options for Questions 63–35:

A Aspirin
B Cisplatin
C Frusemide
D Gentamicin
E Kanamycin
F Neomycin
G Phenytoin
H Propanolol
I Quinine
J Risperidone
K Tobramycin

For each of the following cases, select the single most likely drug responsible. Each option may be used once, more than once or not at all.

63. A 17-year-old girl presents to accident and emergency having taken an overdose. She complains of tinnitus.

64. A 56-year-old man presents with difficulty walking without holding onto something. He also claims that objects bounce up and down when he is in a car. He was recently admitted to hospital and received intravenous treatment for a bladder infection

65. A 21-year-old woman presents with bilateral middle ear effusions. She is generally fit and well, except that she is taking medication for panic attacks, which occur when she is in crowded places such as shopping malls.

Theme: Trauma

Options for Questions 66–67:

A Cerebrospinal fluid leak
B Laryngotracheal injury
C Mandibular fracture
D Oesophageal perforation
E Ossicular discontinuity
F Pinna haematoma
G Temporal bone fracture
H Tympanic perforation

For each of the following cases, select the single most likely injury. Each option may be used once, more than once or not at all.

66. A 35-year-old man presents with an injury to his neck which is associated with hoarseness and stridor.

67. A 15-year-old boy presents with an injury to his ear whilst playing rugby. It is swollen, painful and is boggy to the touch.

Theme: TNM staging

Options for Questions 68–69:

A T1N0M0
B T1N1M0
C T1N1aM0
D T1N1bM0
E T2N0M0
F T2N1M0
G T3N0M0

H T3N1M0
I T4N0M0
J T4N1M0

For each of the following cases, select the single most appropriate TNM stage. Each option may be used once, more than once or not at all.

68. A 45-year-old Chinese woman presents with epistaxis. Examination and biopsy reveals a nasopharyngeal carcinoma confined to the nasopharynx with no palpable neck nodes.

69. A 45-year-old Chinese woman presents with epistaxis. Examination and biopsy reveals a nasopharyngeal carcinoma that extends into the nasal cavity and oropharynx. There is a unilateral neck node measuring 6cm in greatest dimension, above the supraclavicular fossa.

Theme: Facial pain

Options for Questions 70–71:

A Dental pain
B Erysipelas
C Herpes zoster
D Migraine
E Ramsay Hunt Syndrome
F Sinonasal tumour
G Sinusitis
H Temporal arteritis
I Trigeminal neuralgia

For each of the following cases, select the single most likely diagnosis. Each option may be used once, more than once or not at all.

70. A 78-year-old woman presents with tinnitus, headache, jaw claudication and diplopia. Her blood test reveals a raised ESR.

71. A 35-year-old man presents with an acute facial pain. He also describes a preceding aura of flashing lights and has had a number of similar episodes in the past.

Theme: Syndromes

Options for Questions 72–74:

A Burning mouth
B CHARGE
C Cystic fibrosis
D Kartagener's
E Osler–Weber–Rendu syndrome
F Pierre Robin
G Young's

For each of the following cases, select the single most likely syndrome. Each option may be used once, more than once or not at all.

72. A 29-year-old childless male presents complaining of recurrent sinusitis. Investigations reveal obstructive azoospermia and bronchiectasis, but normal ciliary motility.

73. An 8-year-old girl presents with bilateral nasal polyps.

74. A 21-year-old man presents with recurrent sinusitis. Investigations reveal situs inversus and immotile cilia.

Theme: Paediatric airway obstruction

Options for Questions 75–78:

A Acute epiglottitis
B Acute laryngotracheobronchitis (croup)
C Acute tonsillitis
D Allergic reaction
E Choanal atresia
F Chronic obstructive airway disease
G Down syndrome
H Foreign body
I Laryngeal papillomatosis
J Laryngomalacia
K Nasal masses
L Pyriform aperture stenosis
M Severe rhinitis
N Vocal cord palsy

For each of the following cases, select the single most likely diagnosis. Each option may be used once, more than once or not at all.

75. A 3-month-old boy presents with gradually worsening noisy breathing, which is especially noticeable when he eats or is supine. He is on a lower centile for weight gain and has poor food intake.

76. A 4-year-old boy presents with sudden onset noisy breathing and drooling. The child appears scared,

flushed and stridulous. He is pyrexial and using accessory muscles during respiration.

77. An 18-month-old boy presents with a brief history of choking and cyanosis for about 10 seconds, for a few hours earlier. He is now completely asymptomatic.

78. A 7-year-old girl presents with a history of a hoarse voice for around 4 weeks presents with worsening stridor over the last 72 hours. There is no pyrexia. This has been her third admission in just over a year with a similar problem.

Theme: Otological diagnosis

Options for Questions 79–82:

A Acoustic neuroma
B Cholesteatoma
C Chronic serous otitis media
D Impacted wax
E Otitis externa
F Otitis media
G Otosclerosis
H Otospongiosis
I Otosyphilis

For each of the following cases, select the single most likely diagnosis. Each option may be used once, more than once or not at all.

79. A 54-year-old man presents with several months of pungent discharge from his right ear. Otoscopy reveals an attic perforation, combined with a dark brown wax-like material

80. A 60-year-old woman presents with unilateral deafness and tinnitus for many years. On examination, there is an absent corneal reflex and ataxia

81. A 24-year-old man presents with pain in his right ear. On examination there is pus in the external ear canal, which appears, erythematous and swollen.

82. A 55-year-old woman presents with reduced hearing and otalgia in her left ear after spending and evening in a jacuzzi.

Theme: Congenital abnormalities

Options for Questions 83–86:

A Bat/prominent ears
B Canal atresia
C Choanal atresia
D Cleft palate
E Microtia
F Preauricular sinus
G Submucous cleft
H Tracheal stenosis
I Tracheal web
J Tracheomalacia

For each of the following cases, select the single most likely congenital abnormality. Each option may be used once, more than once or not at all.

83. A 1-year-old boy presents with expiratory stridor. There was no history of foreign body inhalation or asthma. Microlaryngoscopy and bronchoscopy reveals a partial obstruction within the lumen of the trachea.

84. A 20-year-old Down syndrome male presents with difficulty breathing. Suspicious of a foreign body, a rigid bronchoscopy is performed, and the trachea is

seen to collapse (with the patient breathing spontaneously. No foreign body is found.

85. A 5-year-old boy presents with bilateral absence of anti-helicies.

86. A 12-year old girl presents with a bifid uvula.

Theme: Systemic diseases in otolaryngology

Options for Questions 87–90:

A Cogan's syndrome
B HIV
C Leprosy
D Polyarteritis nodosa
E Relapsing polychondritis
F Sjögren's syndrome
G Syphilis
H Systemic lupus erythematosus
I Tuberculosis
J Wegener's granulomatosis

For each of the following cases, select the single most likely diagnosis. Each option may be used once, more than once or not at all.

87. A 39-year-old woman presents complains of a two-year history of bilateral hearing loss, tinnitus and distortion associated with difficulty discriminating sounds in background noise. She also mentioned sore red eyes requiring hospital treatment. On examination, she had normal ear canals and tympanic membranes. Audiological assessment revealed

bilateral hearing loss at 2 kHz, and a speech audiogram showed optimal discrimination score of 80%.

88. A 19-year-old girl presents with a rash over her face, and joint pain in her hands. Flexible nasoendoscopic examination revealed nasopharyngeal ulceration.

89. A 54-year-old woman presents complaining of a dry eyes and mouth. Examination also revealed ulnar deviation of her fingers.

90. A 50-year-old male immigrant presents with a significant saddle nose deformity and multiple skin lesions.

Theme: Consent

Options for Questions 91–93

A Make patient ward of court
B Obtain consent from next of kin
C Obtain consent from the parent
D Obtain consent from the patient
E Surgery can proceed
F Surgery cannot proceed

For each of the following cases, select the single most appropriate consent. Each option may be used once, more than once or not at all.

91. A 43-year-old man is admitted from a psychiatric ward having ingested a fish bone. The psychiatrist is in agreement that surgical removal is required.

Unfortunately, the patient is unable to give informed consent.

92. An 8-year-old son of a Jehovah's Witness is brought to hospital with a post tonsillectomy bleed. It fails to settle with conservative measures. He requires a transfusion, and return to theatre. Both parents refuse to consent for either.

93. An 84-year-old woman is discovered unconscious at home with a torrential epistaxis, and is subsequently brought to hospital by ambulance. Arrest of the bleed is required in theatre. Her husband expresses his refusal to allow her to go to theatre.

Theme: Rehabilitation of hearing loss

Options for Questions 94-97

A. Behind-the-ear hearing aid
B. Body worn hearing aid
C. Bilateral Cochlear implants
D. Bone anchored hearing aid (on a soft band)
E. Bone anchored hearing aid (with a titanium screw)
F. Bone anchored hearing aid (with magnets)
G. Bone conduction hearing aid
H. Brainstem implants
I. In the ear hearing aid (conchal)
J. In-the-canal hearing aid
K. Middle ear implant
L. No device
M. Unilateral Cochlear implant
N. Vented behind-the-ear hearing aid

For each of the following cases, select the best strategy for rehabilitation of hearing losss. Each option may be used once, more than once or not at all.

94. A 12 month old year old boy presents with suspected hearing loss because of deformed pinnas and abscent ear canals. On examination, he was also noted to have down slanting palpabre fissures.

95. A 2-year-old boy presents with suspected hearing loss due to poor speech development. Radiological investigations reveal the absence of both cochleas.

96. A 12-year-old girl presents with profound sensori-neural hearing loss following meningitis.

97. A 39-year-old man presents complaining of hearing loss. He is a professional surfer and teaches beginners. Pure tone audiometry reveals a right sided conductive hearing loss with threshold of approximately 45 Dbhl, with normal hearing on the left. He is finding it difficult to hear his fellow surfers.

Theme: Statistical testings

Options for Questions 98–100:

A Chi-squared (χ^2) test
B Fisher's exact-test
C Friedman test
D F-test
E Kruskal–Wallis test
F Mann–Whitney U test
G McNemar

H One Sample (paired) Student's t-test
I One-way analysis of variance (ANOVA)
J Pearson's correlation coefficient
K Spearman's rank correlation coefficient
L Two sample (unpaired) Student's t-test
M Two-way analysis of variance (ANOVA)
N Wilcoxon matched pairs test

For each of the following data sets, select the single most suitable statistical test. Each option may be used once, more than once or not at all.

98. To assess the linear analogue scale responses of a group of subjects (n=15) asked to report their perceived pain on 2 consecutive days.

99. To detect any differences between four consultants' assessments of six trainee candidates performing microlaryngoscopy.

100. In a study of pain following tonsillectomy, patients were randomly allocated to receive either an analgesia, or placebo 2 hours pre-operatively. All patients were asked to rate their pain 2 hours after surgery using the scale: 0=no pain, 1=mild, 2=moderate, 3=severe. Analyse the results.

Answer Keys to Chapter 4 EMIs

<table>
<tr><td>1</td><td>C</td><td>CHARGE syndrome<ul><li>Charge syndrome has a reported prevalence of 1 in 12,000. Diagnosis of CHARGE syndrome is made on the basis of clinical findings and CT imaging of the nose.</li><li>Bilateral choanal atresia is a neonatal airway emergency requiring a secured oropharyngeal airway, orogastric tube and early surgical intervention. An echocardiogram is required before surgical correction of the bilateral atresia.
Features include:<ul><li>Coloboma of the eye (80–90% of individuals) a fissure usually in the back of the eye.</li><li>Heart defect a variety of defects may occur the most common being a septal defect.</li><li>Atresia</li><li>Retardation of growth/development</li><li>Genital abnormalities</li><li>Ear abnormalities. Short, wide ear with deficient lobe, often protruding, asymmetric. Ossicular malformations.</li></ul></li></ul></td></tr>
</table>

		Sensorineural deafness
2	L	Usher syndrome - This syndrome, along with Cogan's and Refsum's, involves both the ears and eyes. It is characterised by sensorineural hearing loss and progressive retinitis pigmentosa. - Usher's syndrome is one of the most common types of autosomal recessive syndromic hearing loss and there are three distinct types, types 1–3, based on the degree of hearing impairment and vestibular involvement. - It presents initially as non-syndromic hearing loss until the retinitis pigmentosa is diagnosed. - Cogan's syndrome is a rare autoimmune disorder is characterized by recurrent inflammation of the cornea (interstitial keratitis), fever, lethargy, dizziness and sensorineural hearing loss. - Refsum syndrome exists in both adult and infantile forms. It is an autosomal recessive neurological disorder caused by over-accumulation of phytanic acid. Features include cerebellar degeneration, retinitis pigmentosa and sensorineural

		hearing loss cataract and epilepsy.
3	G	Goldenhar Syndrome ➢ This is also known as Oculoauriculovertebral spectrum/Hemifacial microsomia/First and second arch syndrome. It is associated with anomalous development of the first and second branchial arch. ➢ Features include; microtia(variable severity ranging from partial to complete atresia of the auditory canal) and from minor/complete absence of the external ear,(Although the condition is usually unilateral it may occasionally be bilateral but is nearly always asymmetrical, differentiating it from Treacher–Collins), preauricular skin tags or hillocks of tissue (which are in a line between tragus and corner of the mouth), deafness: can be sensorineural or conductive, macrostomia: occasionally with lateral facial clefting, epibulbar dermoid (in which case the acronym Goldenhar syndrome is used), vertebral defects, cardiac defects, renal anomalies and mental retardation (uncommon and

		chromosome analysis should be performed when this is present).
4	B	Apert syndrome ➢ This autosomal dominant congenital disorder is one of the first branchial arch syndromes, characterized by craniosynostosis of the skull and facial bones (premature fusion in utero), congenital fixation of the stapes footplate, cleft palate, saddle nose as well as syndactyl malformations of the hands and feet. ➢ It shares some features with Crouzon's syndrome, which is an autosomal dominant genetic disorder affecting the first branchial arch characterized by premature fusion of the facial bones and skull. ➢ Clinical appearances include brachycephaly, exophthalmos, hypertelorism, parrot beak nose, middle and external ear deformities and a hypoplastic maxilla in contrast to a prognathic mandible. ➢ Apert syndrome is often confused with Alport syndrome which is a hereditary disorder is characterized by glomerulonephritis and bilateral sensorineural hearing loss, the latter of which is not present in infancy and

		develops gradually with age
5	F	Down's syndrome ➢ The incidence of Down's syndrome is 1/600 live births. This condition is caused by the presence of extra genetic material related to the 21st chromosome. ➢ During meiosis for gametogenesis 23 pairs of chromosomes (23 maternally inherited and 23 paternally inherited) are duplicated and then quartered to provide haploid gametes (23 chromosomes). Disjunction occurs twice, first in anaphase meiosis I (separation of maternal and paternal chromosomes) and secondly in anaphase meiosis II (separation of chromosomes into chromatids). ➢ If disjunction does not occur correctly, one gamete will be left with 22 chromosomes and the other with 24. If this non disjunction occurs with chromosome 21 it is called Trisomy 21 or Down's. This type of meiotic defect makes up 95% of the phenotypic Down's syndrome patients. ➢ 3–4% occurs due to a Robertsonian Translocation: During meiosis DNA is swapped between paternal and

		maternal chromosomes to allow for phenotype heterogeneity. That is to say genes from paternal chromosome 21 can be replaced with genes from maternal chromosome 21. However, sometimes this translocation is unbalanced and genes move between different chromosomes. For example genes from chromosome 21 can be inserted into chromosome 14. The eventual gamete may end up with just 1 pair of chromosome 21, but it will also have excess chromosome 21 genetic material (inserted somewhere into chromosome 14 in this example). These patients have fewer phenotypic manifestations. ➢ The final cause of Down's is mosaicism. This accounts for the remainder of patients and symptoms are less frequent. In this type the defect occurs during embryogenesis so not all cell lines are affected. ➢ Symptom constellations and clinical features are generally widely recognized: The facial features and manifestations of which include microgenia, epicanthic eyelid fold, upslanting palpebral fissures, macroglossia, recurrent ear infections

		and hearing loss. There is also an association with subglottic stenosis, absent frontal and sphenoid sinuses in addition to Alzheimer's and leukaemias later in life.
6	G	Moebius syndrome ➢ This is a rare congenital neurological disorder caused by the underdevelopment of the VI and VII cranial nerves. This gives rise to an inability to move the eyes laterally and bilateral complete facial paralysis from birth. Rarely the V and VIII cranial nerves are affected. ➢ Since this baby was born by caesarean section it is unlikely the nerve palsies could have arisen from forceps trauma. ➢ It is associated with external ear deformities, mental retardation and mixed hearing loss. Although patients may walk later, most children with eventually catch up. Speech problems often respond to therapy, but may persist due to impaired mobility of the tongue and mouth. As children get older, the lack of facial expression and an inability to smile may become the dominant visible symptoms. Moebius Syndrome is sometimes

		accompanied by Pierre Robin Syndrome.
7	F	Melkersson–Rosenthal Syndrome ➢ This is a neurological disorder characterized by recurrent facial paralysis, swelling of the upper and lower lips and furrows in the tongue. It is also known as granulomatous cheilitis. There is of presence of lymphoedema and noncaseating granulomas in the lamina propria leading to chronic swelling of the lip. ➢ It can be associated with Crohn's disease and sarcoidosis in rare cases. Onset is in childhood or early adolescence. After recurrent attacks (ranging from days to years in between), swelling may persist and increase, eventually becoming permanent. ➢ Treatment is symptomatic and may include medication therapies with nonsteroidal anti-inflammatory drugs (NSAIDs) and corticosteroids to reduce swelling, as well as antibiotics and immunosuppressants ➢ Surgery may be recommended to relieve pressure on the facial nerves and to reduce swollen tissue, but its effectiveness has not been

		established. Massage and electrical stimulation may also be prescribed. ➢ Melkersson–Rosenthal syndrome may recur intermittently after its first appearance. It can become a chronic disorder. Follow-up care should exclude the development of Crohn's disease or sarcoidosis
8	K	Syphilis ➢ Sabre-shaped tibia is seen in syphilitic patient in the same was as sabre-shaped trachea is seen in relapsing polychondritis. Syphilis is caused by the spirochaete bacterium Treponema pallidum and is primarily transmitted through sexual contact although can be acquired vertically from mother to foetus. ➢ It is associated with several forms: primary, secondary, latent, tertiary and congenital. Facial palsy may occur as part of neurosyphilis which is mostly associated with the tertiary form and as such may occur several years or even decades after primary infection. ➢ Primary syphilis involves a single chancre (a firm, painless, non-itchy skin ulceration). It occurs 3–90 days from infection.

		➤ Secondary syphilis occurs ten weeks after infection and involves a diffuse rash which frequently involves the palms of the hands and soles of the feet. ➤ Tertiary syphilis occurs 3–15 years after infection and involves gummas, neurological, or cardiac symptoms. ➤ Diagnosis can be made through the VDRL which has high sensitivity but low specificity. It is usually confirmed with fluorescent treponema antibody absorption.
9	H	Multiple sclerosis ➤ This is a rare central cause of facial palsy due to demyelination of the cranial nerve sheath. It is more common in women and frequently occurs in the 3rd–4th generation of life. ➤ Diagnosis is clinical, but can be aided by MRIs which show two or more central nervous system lesions spread over time and anatomy. ➤ The condition predominantly causes demyelination of nerves in the central nervous system. Common presenting symptoms include loss of vision from optic neuritis and double vision when the medial longitudinal

		fasciculus (connection of 3rd and 6th cranial nerves allowing conjugate gaze) is affected. The condition can be progressive, but more commonly has a relapsing remitting course. ➢ Treatment is with steroids during exacerbations and beta interferon as a disease modifying agent. It should be considered in the differential of a young lady with vertigo as well as facial palsy.
10	B	Heerfordt syndrome ➢ Heerfordt syndrome or uveoparotid fever was first described by an ophthalmologist in 1909. It consists of uveitis, parotitis, fever, and facial nerve palsy. It is thought to be part of the extrapulmonary manifestations of sarcoidosis, however, its incidence in patients with sarcoidosis is 0.3%. 15% of patients with this condition have a close relative with it. ➢ Spontaneous remission usually occurs although treatment should be directed towards underlying sarcoidosis. Anterior uveitis presents with blind spots and painful red eye. Parotitis should be investigated with ultrasound guided biopsy to rule out underlying lymphoma.

		➢ Other ENT manifestations of sarcoidosis include audiovestibular neuropathy from neurosarcoidosis, upper airway deposits causing stridor and sinonasal deposits leading to septal perforations, nasal blockage and epistaxis.
11	F	Labyrinthitis ➢ Acute onset of nausea vomiting and nystagmus is most likely due to labyrinthitis. It occurs when bacterial toxins and host inflammatory mediators, such as cytokines, enzymes, and complement, cross the round window membrane, causing inflammation of the labyrinth in the absence of direct bacterial contamination. ➢ This condition is associated with acute upper respiratory tract infection or chronic middle ear disease and is believed to be one of the most common complications of otitis media. Inflammation of the whole labyrinth leads to a reduction in hearing as well as severe vertigo whereas vestibular neuronitis causes only vertigo. Both conditions are self resolving and can be treated in the acute phase with anti-emetics, rest

		and fluids. The condition can last up to a month. However, frequently following an infection a degree of disequilibrium remains. ➢ Vestibular rehabilitation for these patients has proven beneficial. Irritative activation of the labyrinth causes the eyes to conjugately move to the opposite direction slowly, which is corrected centrally by rapid eye movement back to the centre (e.g. right sided labyrinthitis causes eye to slowly deviate to left. There is a fast phase of eye movement back to the right. This is the basis of nystagmus in these patients. The fast phase is always described and therefore it is said the patient has right sided nystagmus.)
12	B	Citelli's abscess ➢ A Citelli abscess is derived from a subperiosteal abscess which has spread through the medial aspect of the mastoid into the digastric fossa. ➢ A Bezold abscess refers to one that has tracked inferiorly within sheath of the sternomastoid to form swelling along the anterior border of the muscle. ➢ A Luc's abscess is one that extends

		upwards towards the zygoma. These are all recognised complications of acute otitis media. ➢ Other complications include osteomyelitis, extradural and subdural abscesses, brain abscesses, otitic hydrocephalus, lateral sinus thrombosis, serous and suppurative labyrinthitis and facial nerve palsy especially in patients with congenital dehiscence of the horizontal portion of the facial nerve. ➢ Long term sequelae of acute otitis media include non-suppurative middle ear effusion, high frequency sensorineural hearing loss, tympanic membrane perforation, adhesions, tympanosclerosis, and erosion of the ossicular chain.
13	C	Extradural abscess ➢ The 3-year-old girl most likely has an extradural abscess which is the commonest intracranial abscess complication of otitis media. ➢ Chronic suppurative otitis media (CSOM) is a chronic inflammation of the middle ear and mastoid. World Health Organisation's definitions suggests more than two weeks, however, others contend longer e.g.

		up to six weeks. ➢ Clinical features are recurrent otorrhoea through a tympanic perforation, with conductive hearing loss of varying severity. Spread to the brain may be direct, as in this case, or haematological. ➢ Treatment would involve surgical communication between the abscess cavity and the pneumatised portions of the temporal bone. Granulation tissue should be removed until dura is seen. ➢ When answering a viva question it is always good to have a classification system. Complications of otitis media should be separated into intratemporal and intracranial. Intratemporal complications include mastoiditis, labyrinthitis, labyrinthine fistula, petrous apicitis, and facial paralysis. Intracranial complications include meningitis, extradural abscess, intracranial abscess, subdural empyema, sigmoid sinus thrombosis and otitic hydrocephalus.
14	E	Goitre ➢ Goitre is a non-specific term that is used to describe any enlargement of the thyroid. It comes from the Latin

		term gutter which means throat. The commonest cause of a goitre is insufficient thyroxine production to meet demands. This may occur because of inefficient manufacturing process or increased demand. In response to this supply-demand discrepancy the thyroid increases in size to supply more thyroxine, a process governed by excess TSH. Occasionally an area of the gland increases out of proportion to the rest of the thyroid and produces a dominant nodule in a multinodular goitre. ➢ Treatment with thyroxine can slow, arrest and occasionally reverse the goitrogenic process and should be considered in all patients who are hypothyroid, clinically or subclinically. If this fails to reduce the size of the thyroid and there are aerodigestive compression symptoms then surgery (total thyroidectomy) can be considered. ➢ For examination purposes classification of the causes of goitres is given below: ➢ Physiological: Puberty -increased metabolic

		demand Pregnancy -increased demand; increased TBG Physiologic stress of any kind ➢ Autoimmune: Graves' disease Hashimoto's thyroiditis ➢ Thyroiditis: Subacute granulomatous / de Quervain's Subacute lymphocytic / silent Riedel's thyroiditis - uncommon; gland usually shrinks Acute infective -transient Infiltrative e.g. sarcoidosis, tuberculosis ➢ Iodine deficiency -simple, endemic goitre ➢ Idiopathic -simple, sporadic goitre ➢ Multinodular goitre -develops from simple goitre ➢ Dyshormonogenesis -including Pendred syndrome: ➢ Inability to use trapped iodine ➢ Deficiency of peroxidase and dehalogenase ➢ Abnormal protein binding in the plasma

		➢ Goitrogens ➢ Thyroid cysts -rare ➢ Thyroid tumours
15	B	Cervical rib ➢ A cervical rib usually developments from seventh cervical vertebra. It occurs in 1 in 200 people. The cervical rib may be bony and attached to the first normal rib, its cartilage or the sternum. It may project freely with no anterior attachment. ➢ Alternatively, it may be a thin, fibrous strand which paradoxically may produce more symptoms than a complete rib. In half the cases, it is unilateral, usually on the right side. ➢ The subclavian artery and first thoracic nerve may be affected as they pass over the cervical rib to gain access to the upper limb. The artery may be narrowed, with post-stenotic dilatation. Thrombus may collect in this aneurysm, predisposing to emboli and acute ischaemia. The nerve may be damaged by direct pressure. ➢ A cervical rib is a common cause of the thoracic outlet syndrome. Excessive use of the arms can cause blood to be diverted around the

		blockage from anastomoses around the common carotid and therefore relative lack of blood to the brain leading to loss of consciousness and occasionally transient ischaemic attacks. This is called subclavian steal syndrome. ➢ Surgery should be considered for symptomatic patients.
16	J	Subclavian artery aneurysm ➢ The subclavian artery starts comes off the aortic arch on the left and the brachiocephalic trunk on the right. It becomes the axillary artery as it crosses the outer edge of the first thoracic rib. It supplies blood to the shoulder, arm, forearm and hand on its ipsilateral side. ➢ A true aneurysm is an unnatural dilatation of all three layers of an artery. A false aneurysm refers to thrombus around the artery, giving the impression of vessel dilatation. Aneurysms are felt clinically by expansile pulsatile masses. ➢ True subclavian artery aneurysms are relatively rare lesions. Thoracic outlet compression is responsible for 75% of aneurysms. They are formed as a result of compression by for example

		a cervical rib. A subclavian aneurysm can cause compression on local veins and nerves, causing deep vein thrombosis and neuropathies, respectively. Thrombus forms within an aneurysm and can cause distal embolisation.
17	H	Pharyngeal pouch ➢ The history and characteristics of the lump suggest that the patient has a pharyngeal pouch. This condition is more common in European Caucasians and rare in Japanese and Indonesians. It has a male:female ratio of 1.5:1. It is almost completely confined to those over 60 ➢ The underlying pathophysiology is thought to be tight cricopharyngeus muscle, or inability of the muscle to relax in a coordinated fashion during pharyngeal phase of swallow. This may be secondary to laryngopharyngeal reflux. Pressure builds up proximal to the tight cricopharyngeus. There is a weakness in the musculature between the oblique fibres of the inferior constrictor and the transverse fibres of cricopharyngeus. Pressure in these areas causes a pulsion diverticulum

		through the area of weakness. There is more space on the left due to the laterally placed carotid and the left cervical oesophageal curvature. Hence 90% of pouches are on the left side. ➢ Symptoms include dysphagia with regurgitation of undigested foods and aspiration leading to recurrent pneumonias. ➢ Investigations for diagnosis include barium swallow. Further direct visualisation should be undertaken to exclude the possibility of a pouch tumour. ➢ Treatment can be conservative with change in diet and speech and language referral. However, for recalcitrant cases endoscopic stapling of the pouch can be considered. This procedure requires good peroral access to the pharynx. ➢ Unfortunately this patient age group often has cervical osteoarthrosis limiting neck extension. When patients have their own teeth access is more difficult and fraught with the possibility of dental damage. If endoscopic surgery fails, open surgery can be performed. However,

		this is an operation with considerable comorbidity and the possibility of leak and fistulisation. Endoscopic surgery should focus on dividing the bar that separates the oesophagus from the pouch to make one lumen. ➢ Open surgery involves excision of the pouch and division of cricopharyngeus to alleviate the underlying pathology.
18	A	Branchial cyst ➢ The position and feature of the lump is typical of a branchial cyst. Since branchial cysts are lined by squamous epithelial tissue and contain lymphoid tissue, they are thought to arise from squamous epithelial rests within lymph nodes, during embryological development. ➢ Other theories suggest that they arise from remnants of the first pharyngeal pouch, cervical sinus or thymic duct of the third pharyngeal pouch. ➢ Always consider that a 'branchial cyst' may be a degenerated lymph node squamous cell metastatic deposit in anyone over 40 and obtain the appropriate FNA and imaging before potentially oncologically jeopardising the neck by an ill considered incision.

19	G	Sulcus vocalis ➢ The aetiology of sulcus vocalis is unknown. It is a linear scar in the free of the true vocal cord tethered to the lamina propria. It therefore, prevents a free mucosal wave. It can be caused by previous surgery but may also be a de-roofed cyst. It causes the pitch to become higher, which is often unnoticed in women. ➢ Other symptoms include hoarseness, vocal fatigue, voice weakness, and increased effort. ➢ Prevalence is hard to determine. Necropsy studies show some degree of sulcus on 20% of patients. ➢ Diagnosis is made on videostroboscopy which shows an area of non-movement during phonation. ➢ Speech therapy is important for treatment. If this fails then hyaluronic acid injection into the scar to lift it from the lamina propria may be attempted.
20	J	Vocal cord polyp ➢ Voice breaks suggests that the vocal cords are failing to meet. This can be caused by palsy or vocal cord masses (nodules, polyps, granulomas and

		cancer). ➢ There is often a foreign body sensation in the throat with a chronic cough and recurrent throat clearing. ➢ Vocal cord polyps and singer's nodules tend to be in the middle of the vocal cord whereas granulomas are based posteriorly. Nodules are bilateral by definition, whereas polyps and granulomas can be unilateral or bilateral. ➢ Singer's nodules are rare in adult males and should be investigated further. ➢ Granulomas are often related to phontrauma and laryngopharyngeal reflux. ➢ Polyps can be treated with speech therapy but normally go on to surgery for excision. Care should be taken to preserve the free mucosal edge of the vocal cord.
21	I	Vocal cord palsy ➢ Left vocal cord palsy is more common than right due to the long tortuous course of the left recurrent laryngeal nerve that traverses into the mediastinum before looping around the arch of the aorta to return into the neck.

		➢ To generate voice with a permanently abducted vocal cord requires overcompensation from the functioning cord and a more powerful expiration. Hence these patients often get winded when speaking and sound dyspnoeic. ➢ When investigating vocal cord palsy it is important to know the anatomy of the vagus and the recurrent laryngeal nerve. The RLN is a branch of the vagus and is a myelinated nerve. It sits anteriorly amongst vagal nerve fibres as the vagus leaves the medulla. As the vagus descends it rotates medially. The vagus leaves the skull via the jugular foramen and has a superior ganglion just before it exits. Tumours of the jugular foramen can affect some vagal fascicles whilst others are left intact. In the neck the vagus travels in the carotid sheath. The left vagus nerve crosses anterior to the aortic arch. The RLN arising from the vagal nerve just below the aortic arch loops medially under the aorta and ascends within the tracheoesophageal groove. The right vagus nerve gives off the right RLN at the level of division of the innominate

		artery. At this point the right RLN loops around the subclavian artery and ascends along the superior lobe of the pleura. It then approaches the tracheoesophageal groove behind the common carotid artery. ➢ The approximate length of the left recurrent laryngeal nerve is 12 cm, where as the right nerve measures 6 cm. The right recurrent laryngeal nerve does not get into the tracheoesophageal groove until it approaches the cricothyroid joint. In some patients the right recurrent laryngeal nerve is given off from the vagus nerve at the level of thyroid gland, which is always associated with an anomalous retroesophageal location of the right subclavian artery. ➢ One third of RLN palsies are idiopathic, one third iatrogenic (e.g. after thyroidectomy and oesophagectomy) and one third related to tumours. Examination should rule out glottis, subglottic and hypopharyngeal cancers as a possible cause. Imaging should follow the course of the nerve from the skull base to the larynx, which would

		involve the imaging the chest if the left RLN is involved. ➢ Treatment involves speech therapy and if this fails surgery can be considered. Surgery focuses on medicalisation of the abducted vocal cord. This can be done via injection of material (Bioplastique/fat) or by medialisation thyroplasty (Ishiki procedures). A newer option includes re-innervation of the larynx.
22	F	Spasmodic dysphonia ➢ This condition is most common in women in the 40's. There are three main types of spasmodic dysphonia: Abductor and Adductor. They are both considered to be neurological conditions with familial tendencies. They are also called laryngeal dystonias. ➢ The adductor subtype causes spasms of over adduction during speech. This causes the voice to sound strangled and strained. The disease is task specific and therefore has no affect on swallowing or muscles of supraglottis. In fact it is difficult to replicate the findings during laughter and singing (although singers do have reduced ability to hit certain notes).

		➢ Abductor dysphonia causes the vocal cords to spasm open and therefore prevents a mucosal wave. These patients have a weak breathy voice. Essential tremor is persistent through all tasks and often has associated tremor of the tongue. The frequency of tremor is 12 Hz. Patients often whisper to mask the tremor. ➢ Treatment for both can include Botox injections.
23	C	Petrotympanic fissure. ➢ The chorda tympani is third branch of the facial nerve is concerned with taste in the anterior two thirds of the tongue as well secretomotor function for the submandibular gland. ➢ It enters the temporal bone through the internal auditory canal as part of the facial nerve. It runs posterior to anterior through the middle ear on the medial side of the malleus. It exits through the petrotympanic fissure into the infratemporal fossa. It joins the lingual nerve, a branch of the mandibular division of the trigeminal nerve. The facial nerve exits the skull via the internal auditory meatus and enters the temporal bone. As it exits the auditory meatus it gives off the

		greater superficial petrosal nerve. ➢ The intralabyrinthine portion heads anteriorly towards the geniculate ganglion. At the ganglion the nerve turns back on itself and heads posteriorly (known as the tympanic portion). As the nerve enters the mastoid it changes direction to head inferiorly known as the descending portion. It exits the mastoid at the stylomastoid foramen.
24	K	Tensor tympani. ➢ Tensor tympani is contained in a bony canal above the osseous part of the Eustachian tube. It originates at the osseocartilaginous junction of the Eustachian tube and the adjoining part of the greater wing of the sphenoid bone as well as the osseous canal. ➢ It enters the middle ear and makes a sharp bend around a septum known as processus cochleariformis and inserts into the manubrium of the malleus. It is thought that its function is to dampen sounds from chewing. ➢ Patients with hyperacusis may have an increased activity in the tensor tympani muscle as part of the startle response to some sounds.

		➢ It is innervated by the nerve to medial pterygoid which is a branch of the mandibular division of the trigeminal nerve and is a derivative of the first branchial pouch.
25	F	Pyramidal eminence. ➢ The stapedius muscle is a derivative of the 2nd branchial pouch is the smallest muscle in the body and is housed in the pyramidal eminence. The tendon exits from a little foramen in the prominence and inserts into stapes neck. ➢ Nerve supply is from the second division of the facial nerve. Its function is to reduce noise from your own voice getting to through the oval window. It can reduce transduction of sound by 20bD when activated. Tensor tympani has a similar function, but to reduce the transmission of mastication sounds to the ear. ➢ The stapedial reflex is the stiffening of the stapes in response to a loud sound. It can be used to check the integrity of the facial nerve and also to help diagnose otosclerosis and auditory neuropathies.

26	G	Scutum ➢ The scutum is a sharp bony spur formed by the lateral wall of the tympanic cavity and the superior wall of the external auditory canal. Retraction of the pars flaccida into the epitympanum causes pressure on the scutum and causes erosion. ➢ Scutum and ossicular erosion are sensitive markers for cholesteatoma on a CT scan. Therefore the scutum is a landmark of radiological significance and not surgical. ➢ Prussak's space is a region in the epitympanum where cholesteatomas occur. It is of radiological significance. It is medially bounded by the neck of the malleus and laterally bounded by the pars flaccida. ➢ Both the scutum and Prussak's space are markers used to help make the diagnosis of cholesteatoma on a CT scan. However, CT should not be used to diagnose cholesteatoma as it is a clinical diagnosis.
27	H	Sinus tympani ➢ The sinus tympani is an anatomical area that lies between the labyrinthine wall and the pyramidal

		process. It is located in the posterior tympanic cavity and is an area difficult to approach or visualize. ➢ It is essentially a posterior extension of the mesotympanum, inaccessible surgically because of the posterior semicircular canal. Hence it is a frequent site of residual and recurrent cholesteatoma. Mirrors and endoscopes have been used to visualise the area to ensure full removal of the cholesteatoma. ➢ The facial recess is the area between the tympanic annulus and the pyramidal process. Opening this area gives better access to ensure all cholesteatoma is removed.
28	D	Mikulicz's syndrome ➢ Comprises chronic bilateral hypertrophy of the lacrimal, parotid and salivary glands, associated with chronic lymphocytic infiltration. Patients usually have a narrowing of the palpebral fissures and a parchment-like dry mouth. It is regarded as a clinical variant of Sjogren's syndrome. ➢ In a patient with painful parotid swellings, questions should be asked about sicca syndrome. These patients

		can be diagnosed with Schirmers test and anti-rho/la antibodies. Ultrasound is helpful and biopsy is occasionally needed. But excision is rarely necessary. ➢ Treatment of underlying Sjorgrens often helps the parotitis.
29	I	Warthin's tumour ➢ Also known as papillary cystadenoma lymphomatosum or adenolymphoma, it is a benign tumour generally affects the parotid glands, primarily in the tail. ➢ It accounts for around 5% of all parotid tumours. 10% of these tumours occur bilaterally. It usually occurs after middle age and has a strong male preponderance with a male: female ratio of 5:1. There is a notable association with smoking. ➢ Some Warthin's tumours have been reported outside of the parotid in lymph nodes or in tissue just adjacent to the parotid. A typical Warthin's tumour is encapsulated, smooth, and lobular. Microscopically, there are papillary formations, cystic spaces and a supporting stroma of dense lymphoid tissue with follicles. The lymphoid tissue is a reactive

		component.
30	G	Ranula ➢ Latin word rana, meaning 'frog' are mucoceles that occur in the floor of the mouth and usually involve the major salivary glands. The ranula originates in the body of the sublingual gland, in the ducts of Rivini of the sublingual gland, in the Wharton duct of the submandibular gland, and occasionally from the minor salivary glands at this location. ➢ They are divided into two types: oral and cervical/plunging ranulas. Oral ranulas are secondary to mucus extravasation that pools superior to the mylohyoid muscle, whereas cervical ranulas are associated with mucus extravasation along the fascial planes of the neck. ➢ The main operative risk is to the lingual nerve. Simple marsupuilisation in this case is not sufficient and formal exploration and excision is necessary.
31	I	Squamous cell carcinoma ➢ Squamous cell carcinoma of the skin arises from the epidermal layer. It is a histologically distinct form of cancer arising from the uncontrolled

		multiplication of cells of epithelium, or cells showing particular cytological or tissue architectural characteristics of squamous cell differentiation, such as the presence of keratin, tonofilament bundles, or desmosomes. ➢ SCC of the skin begins as a small nodule and as it enlarges the centre becomes necrotic and sloughs and the nodule turns into an ulcer. Unlike basal cell carcinoma (BCC), squamous cell carcinoma (SCC) has a substantial risk of metastasis especially in SCC arising in scars, on the lower lips or mucosa, and occurring in immunosuppressed patients. ➢ About one-third of lingual and mucosal tumors metastasise before diagnosis (these are often related to tobacco and alcohol use).
32	C	Chondrodermatits nodularis helicis ➢ This is more common in middle aged men who have sustained injury to the pinna. The poor blood supply to the region in addition to repeated trauma is thought to precipitate a localised chondritis. ➢ Clinically it presents with a sudden appearance of a painful nodule on

		the helix or antihelix on sun damaged skin that has recently suffered trauma. The nodule may rapidly increase in size until it reaches a stable maximum. ➢ Treatment includes avoid pressure on the area, topical antibiotics, intralesional steroids and surgical excision. ➢ Differential diagnosis for a new lesion appearing in an area of sun damaged skin should always include basal cell carcinoma and squamous cell carcinoma. If in doubt excision biopsy should be undertaken. ➢ Wedge excisions or primary excision and Wolfe graft allow for large excisions with safe margins and minimal cosmetic impact.
33	G	Relapsing polychondritis ➢ This is an autoimmune condition with the underlying pathophysiology thought to be auto-antibodies to cartilage specific collagen type II. Patients often have other associated autoimmune conditions like the seronegative arthritides. Occasionally it is a paraneoplastic manifestation of a haematological malignancy. ➢ The swelling always spares the lobule

differentiating it from pinna cellulitis. Nasal septal cartilage and tracheal cartilage is commonly affected, producing stridor and saddling of the nasal bridge.

- Treatment includes steroids, dapsone, azathioprine, and anti-TNF alpha inhibitors.
- Relapsing polychondritis is a rare disorder and the aetiology remains unknown. It is often associated with autoimmune disorders, and the presence of antibodies to type II collagen suggests that it may be immunologically mediated. As it is a rare multisystem disorder with no specific diagnostic test and numerous possible symptoms, a number of diagnostic criteria have been devised. The most widely used are the McAdam's criteria. The following features are sought:
    - Recurrent chondritis of both auricles.
    - Chondritis of nasal cartilages.
    - Chondritis of the respiratory tract, involving laryngeal or tracheal cartilage.
    - Non-erosive inflammatory polyarthritis.

		➢ Inflammation of ocular structures ➢ Cochlear or vestibular damage.
34	H	Sebaceous cyst ➢ A sebaceous cyst develops from a blocked sebaceous gland, which produces sebum that keeps the skin soft and oily. It is sometimes confused with an epidermoid cyst or pilar cyst. ➢ An epidermoid cyst originates in the epidermis and a pilar cyst originates from hair follicles. They contain keratin, a toothpaste-like material. A punctum is seen in 50% of cases which is pathonomic. They are part of the epidermis and only found in areas that are hair-bearing. The area of attachment to the skin prevents the cyst moving independently on physical examination. ➢ An ulcerative infected sebaceous cyst (Cock's peculiar tumour) may mimic a squamous cell carcinoma. Multiple sebaceous cysts are found in an autosomal dominant condition called Gardner's syndrome which is also associated with intestinal hamartomas and osteotomes.

		➢ Treatment can be conservative or surgical. Surgery involves elliptical incision and removal of cyst in toto. Care must be taken not to leave any cyst remnants to avoid recurrence. Surgical excision should not be planned for an acute infection. Incision and drainage can be performed here and surgical excision delayed for 6 weeks.
35	A	Auricular endochondral pseudocyst ➢ This is a condition of unknown aetiology. A defect in auricular embryogenesis, that causes the formation of residual tissue planes, is thought to predispose to the condition. When subjected to repeated minor trauma or mechanical stress, these tissue planes may open, forming a pseudocyst. ➢ Cartilage forms around the pseudocyst. The auricular cartilage is more susceptible due to its lack of connective tissue overlying the cartilage with firm adherence to the skin. This condition is probably on a spectrum of disease shared with an acute perichondrial haematoma. ➢ Treatment is complicated by a cartilaginous covering. Incision and

<table>
<tr><td></td><td></td><td>drainage should be the mainstay with obliteration of the cavity with curette and compression closure.</td></tr>
<tr><td>36</td><td>J</td><td>Stenger's test
➢ This is a tuning fork test for used to differentiate feigned from true unilateral hearing loss. A number of techniques may be employed but on example of using the principle is to present speech or tone stimuli to both ears at a level of 20 dB over threshold in the better ear (and in the worse ear 20 dB below the level of the good ear).
➢ The patient will react as they are able to hear the signal in the better ear. The test continues by increasing the intensity level of the worse ear. If the hearing loss in the worse ear is genuine the patient will keep responding to the signal presented to the better ear (Negative Stenger). If the patient is feigning the hearing impairment they will stop responding when the level of the worse ear exceeds the signal presented to the good ear (Positive Stenger).</td></tr>
<tr><td>37</td><td>C</td><td>The Auditory Response Cradle
➢ This is a fully automated microprocessor controlled machine</td></tr>
</table>

			that was designed for the hearing screening of full term neonates. It monitors behavioural responses to the production of sound. ➢ Head turning, startle responses, body movements and breathing are recorded by pressure transducers in the head rest and mattress. The stimulus is 5 second bursts of sound. The microprocessor makes an objective verdict of pass or fail. This test is rarely used now as is expensive and has been overtaken by new born screening with otoacoustic emissions (OAE). ➢ Cochlea generates its own noise, probably as a result of outer hair cell movement. This is either spontaneous but can also be in response to clicks and is called transient OAE. New born screening uses transient OAE to check hearing status. The test checks the integrity of outer inner, middle ear and cochlea only. When transient OAE are present in response to clicks it suggests that hearing level is at least 40 dB. However, unlike pure tone audiograms, auditory response cradles, distraction tests and auditory

		brain stem evoked responses the integrity of the auditory pathway beyond the cochlea cannot be verified. If a child fails OAE further investigation neecs to be undertaken. ➢ This would include full examination and imaging to ensure no dysplasia/aplasia of the cochlea. If OAEs are present and there are suspicions of reduced hearing further investigations need to be undertaken. These would include full examination, distraction testing/auditory response cradle depending on local facilities and auditory brain stem evoked responses.
38	F	Distraction test ➢ This test was devised by the Ewings in 1944 and over 50 years later is still being modified and usec in clinics and hospitals. The distraction tests is now less utilised because of the introduction of neonatal otoacoustic screening. ➢ Procedure: Two trained testers are required. The baby is seated on the parent/carer's lap facing forward and sitting erect. One tester, the occupier, captures and controls his/her attention by a simple activity with, for

		example a spinning object or small toy on a low table and then covers the object with the baby's hands. The second tester, the distractor, presents the sound stimulus on a horizontal level with the baby's ear at a distance of one metre and at an angle of 45 degrees outside the baby's field of vision. ➢ Commonly, the sounds presented are two high frequency and one low frequency. In a screening programme they are presented at minimal levels (< 35 dBA) and for diagnostic testing the threshold of detectability is measured. 'No sound' trials are used to check for searching behaviour.
39	A	Acoustic reflexes (AR) ➢ These measure the stapedius and tensor tympani reflex generated eardrum movement in response to intense sound. Conventionally it is held that the input to the AR is hearing (VIIIth nerve) and the output is the stapedius muscle (VIIth nerve). There is an ipsilateral and a contralateral pathway. ➢ Ordinarily, there is no consideration made of the tensor tympani's contribution to the AR, although it is

		a similar reflex but mediated through the Vth cranial nerve rather than the VIIth cranial nerve. The contralateral pathway goes in to the VIIIth nerve and synapses in the cochlear nucleus, but then is transferred across the trapezoid body to the superior olive, and then to the VIIth nerve nucleus and stapedius. ➢ Patterns of Acoustic Reflexes Scaling of reflexes. Reflexes are ordinarily present for fairly loud sounds, relative to hearing ability. Usually a 70–90 dB sound is required to produce an AR in a normal hearing individual, or a person with a mild to moderate cochlear hearing loss. ➢ Reflexes may be absent even to louder inputs in patients with: Conductive hearing loss; Otosclerosis, or other middle ear disease. Stapes fixation in probe ear Severe sensory hearing loss VIIIth nerve hearing loss (e.g. an acoustic neuroma) VIIth nerve injury on side being measured.
40	G	7 episodes (per year) ➢ The following are recommended as

		indications for consideration of tonsillectomy for recurrent acute sore throat in both children and adults: (SIGN guidelines) ➢ Sore throats are due to acute tonsillitis ➢ The episodes of sore throat are disabling and prevent normal functioning ➢ Seven or more well documented, clinically significant, adequately treated sore throats in the preceding year or ➢ Five or more such episodes in each of the preceding two years or ➢ Three or more such episodes in each of the preceding three years.
41	B	2 episodes ➢ There are many considerations for tonsillectomy. Cancer and quinsy is amongst the stronger indications. Severe tonsillitis severe enough to hospitalise patients is a very good reason to have the tonsils removed and the ENT UK positional paper on the matter suggests that patients who had even one episode of quinsy

		may consider surgical removal of tonsils within the year. However, most authorities use two episodes of quinsies as to list a patient for surgical management. ➢ As the rate of tonsillectomy in the country is reducing the rate of hospital admissions for tonsillectomy and quinsies has increased. The increasing burden on state suggests we may be underperforming tonsillectomy. However, an overall cost analysis has not been undertaken. ➢ There are two possible pathogenetic mechanisms to the formation of quinsy: Infection of the tonsil progresses through the crypta magna, past the tonsil capsule and causes peritonsillar cellulitis. This then progresses to necrosis and abscess formation in the plane between the tonsil capsule and the superior constrictor. This mechanism is enabled by multiple previous attacks of tonsillitis which have cause obliteration of the intertonsillar clefts. ➢ The second proposed mechanism involves Webers salivary ducts. These

		salivary ducts drain to the tonsil and aid in removal of debris that is caught in tonsil crypts. However, if the ducts are blocked the glands become swollen and can necrose leading to abscess formation. This theory is supported by occurrences of quinsy in patients who have had a tonsillectomy.
42	D	Langerhans cells ➢ A Langerhans cell is a multinucleated giant cell formed by the fusion of activated macrophages and is typically seen in granulomatous diseases such as sarcoidosis and tuberculosis. It has a large central cytoplasmic mass and numerous peripherally arranged nuclei. ➢ In contrast, Langerhans' cell is an antigen-presenting cell found in the skin. ➢ Mikulicz's cells are the activated macrophages seen in rhinoscleroma whilst Russell's bodies are eosinophilic round structures associated with plasma cells seen in the same condition. ➢ Schaumann's bodies are found in sarcoid granulomas together with asteroids.

43	I	Reed–Sternberg cells ➢ Hodgkin's disease is characterised by the neoplastic proliferation of an atypical form of lymphoid cells known as Reed–Sternberg. It is a binucleated cell, resembling owl's eye and shows CD15 and CD 30 positivity. ➢ Warthin–Finkeldey giant cells are found in lymphoid tissue with measles. ➢ Hodgkin's lymphoma commonly presents with cervical lymphadenopathy. There is a painless rapid enlargement of lymph nodes, which are felt to be rubbery on examination. Other symptoms include cyclical high grade fever (Pel–Ebstein fever) weight loss, night sweats and pain in lymph nodes on alcohol consumption. The disease is grouped according to histology of the lymph nodes and then staged according to disease extend by Ann Arbour classification.
44	A	Haller cells. ➢ These refer to an infraorbital ethmoidal air cell that extends along the medial roof of the maxillary sinus.

		Haller cells may cause narrowing to the infundibulum, if they are large. ➢ The goal of functional endoscopic sinus surgery is to improve drainage of the sinuses into natural channels. There is debate as to on how wide antrostomies should be made. Previously wide opening of the sinuses into the nose were recommended. However, there has been a shift towards smaller opening to prevent nitrous oxide washout (which helps mucosa stay healthy). ➢ A Haller cell may limit drainage from the maxillary sinus into the infundibulum despite large antrostomy. Therefore, scans should be carefully examined pre-operatively. Haller cells, unless recognised, may also lead a surgeon to inadvertently enter the orbit. If there is maxillary sinus disease it is recommended that the Haller cell be opened up.
45	H	Onodi cells. ➢ These air cells are lateral and posterior extension of the ethmoid air cells and are also known as the sphenoethmoidal cells. They may surround the optic nerve tracts and

<table>
<tr><td></td><td></td><td>are therefore important in sinus surgery. Unless recognised they can lead to inadvertent damage of the optic nerve.
➢ Although the eponymous names of these cells are unimportant, it is vital to grasp the anatomical principles of sinus surgery. For instance there are variations of middle turbinate and uncinate insertions superiorly that have a profound effect on surgical planning.
➢ The sphenoid can be entered directly from the nasal cavity in-between the septum and the middle turbinate. The natural os is seen here and can be widened. The sphenoid can also be entered from the posterior ethmoid air cells. The carotid artery as well as the optic nerve runs indent on the sphenoid and should be avoided by careful planning.</td></tr>
<tr><td>46</td><td>F</td><td>Michaels's bodies
➢ The origin of congenital cholesteatoma is thought to be due to the persistence of a nest of cells (epidermoid formation) in the middle ear. It was re-discovered by L Michaels at University College London.</td></tr>
</table>

		<ul><li>Congenital cholesteatoma presents in pediatric population with conductive hearing loss and occasionally otalgia.</li><li>Examination shows an intact tympanic membrane with a pearly white lesion behind the membrane. There usually is little history of previous ear infections.</li><li>Congenital cholesteatoma has a predilection for anterosuperior tympanic cavity superior to the eustachian tube orifice.</li><li>If left untreated the cholesteatoma will grow like an acquired cholesteatoma and can lead to intracranial extension.</li><li>Imaging is required to determine the anatomy of the disease which occasionally can extend into the petrous apex.</li></ul>
47	C	Endemic goitre<ul><li>This is due to iodine deficiency and as such is rare in the UK due to treatment of water sources. However, globally it is the most prevalent cause of goitre.</li><li>Deficiency of iodine results in reduced levels of thyroxine and triiodothyronine. Thyroid epithelium hyperplasia occurs due to an increase</li></ul>

		in TSH levels from feedback pathways. ➢ Treatment can be done through thyroxine and dietary supplementation. If this fails and there are aerodigestive compressive symptoms a total thyroidectomy can be considered. ➢ For all patients with a thyroid swelling thyroid function tests and ultrasound should be done as a minimum. If there are signs of a dominant nodule then fine needle aspiration cytology should be undertaken.
48	E	Follicular carcinoma ➢ This is the second most common cause of cancer of the thyroid after papillary. It is a well-differentiated encapsulated tumour that is characterised by haematogenous spread e.g. lung. ➢ Fine-needle aspiration is unable to differentiate between adenoma and carcinoma. Therefore a more definitive biopsy is required – usually a lobectomy. ➢ It is important to understand the THY classification of these cancers: THY1 inadequate; THY2 benign; THY3 indeterminate; THY4 suspicious; THY5

		malignant. ➢ Follicular lesions are classically defined as Thy3 and a diagnostic lobectomy is undertaken. If it is an adenoma then no further treatment need ensue. If carcinoma is found the size of the mass and the age of the patient need to be considered. Completion thyroidectomy can be undertaken for the large tumours. ➢ Newer staging systems include thy3a (malignant) and thy3b (benign) based on histological findings. The use of these subclassifications in surgical planning is yet undefined.
49	I	Medullary carcinoma ➢ This carcinoma originates from the parafollicular C-cells of the thyroid gland (originally derived from the ultimobranchial body of the 4th branchial pouch). ➢ It can present as an isolated neck lump. The associated lymphadenopathy is common finding. ➢ Medullary carcinoma usually presents later in life, can be associated with multiple endocrine neoplasias, MENIIA and MENIIB, it can present much earlier. Calcitonin levels are occasionally used to assess whether

		there is any residual disease after surgery or recurrence. The patient may also have a history suggesting other endocrine dysfunction such phaeochromocytoma.
50	G	Hashimoto's disease ➢ This is part of the spectrum of autoimmune disease and the most common cause of goitrous hypothyroidism in non-iodine deficient areas. ➢ Typically there is aggressive destruction of thyroid cells by various cell-and antibody-mediated immune processes (in contrast to the stimulatory Type V hypersensitivity effect seen in Graves' disease). ➢ It is not yet understood why this occurs but antiperoxidase antibodies are involved. Triggers suggested include iodine, medications, infection, smoking and possibly stress. ➢ The individual usually presents with symptoms of hypothyroidism with/without neck swelling. ➢ The characteristic histological features include a diffuse lymphocytic and plasma cell infiltration with formation of lymphoid follicles and

		thyroid parenchymal atrophy. ➢ Treatment is with thyroid hormone replacement as the patient eventually becomes hypothyroid after the initial hyperthyroid phase.
51	D	HB Grade IV. ➢ In House–Brackmann grade IV this is moderate to severe dysfunction of the facial nerve with obvious weakness and/or disfiguring asymmetry. There is no forehead movement, incomplete eye closure and asymmetry at the angles of mouth. However at rest, tone and symmetry are normal. ➢ House–brackmann is just one of the many facial nerve grading systems. If you are unsure of the grade it is important to document the individual muscle function outcomes. ➢ The original HB score was devised to score post acoustic neuroma facial nerve injury. When a patient with facial nerve palsy is seen it is important to classify whether it is upper or lower motor neurone. Generally speaking if the forehead is surprisingly unaffected in comparison to the rest of the lower face the upper motor neurone causes should

		be considered. This is due to bi cortical representation of the frontalis.
52	B	HB Grade II. ➢ In contrast to House–Brackmann III, grade II is characterised by only slight weakness of the facial nerve, noticeable on close inspection. There is complete eye closure with effort in both grades but grade II has moderate to good forehead function whilst grade III has slight movement. Grade I is normal facial motor function. ➢ When reviewing a patient with lower motor neurone facial nerve paralysis it is important to exclude all causes first before labelling the patient with Bell's palsy. ➢ Therefore it is important to do a detailed neurological, ontological and head and neck examination first. In addition certain blood tests looking for Lyme disease, sarcoidosis and autoimmune conditions can be considered. MRI scanning of the nerve can also be undertaken if history, examination and initial blood tests point you in the direction of an anatomical derangement.

53	F	HB Grade VI. ➢ This grade describes total facial paralysis with no movements at all. The worse the presenting grade the worse the prognosis. Patients with grade VI are often left with residual deficit or synkinesis. ➢ When treating a patient with lower motor neurone facial nerve paralysis oral steroids should be started as soon as possible. This has been shown to reduce recovery period and reduce the chance of residual defect. ➢ Preventative treatment of eyes to reduce the chance of corneal ulcers should be a priority. ➢ Use of anti-virals has not been shown to benefit outcome on large meta-analyses. However, there have been good randomised controlled studies that show benefit of valacyclovir in Bell's palsy patients. ➢ If a patient's HB score is not improving at all it may be necessary to investigate them further with imaging if this has not already been done. The minority of these patients will go in to have surgery. However, stratification of their muscle weakness with electromyography

		over time is useful adjunct in deciding who is likely to need surgery in this slow resolving sub set of patients.
54	D	Exostoses ➢ Exostoses are more common in men than women. They tend to occur after repeated exposure to cold water. The water causes a temperature related peri-osteitis and subsequent new bone growth. ➢ They tend to be bilateral and originate from the tympanic bone. They cause symptoms when large enough by producing a conductive hearing loss and preventing the clearance of wax. ➢ They do not need surgical management unless they are causing considerable conductive hearing loss or to improve approach to middle ear. ➢ They are usually an incidental finding and their bony nature can be confirmed by probing under a microscope. ➢ Exostoses are covered by a squamous epithelium with underlying periosteum. The internal structure of the lesion is characterized by parallel concentric dense layers of sub-periosteal bone abundant in osteocytes and devoid of fibro-vascular channels and their contents so characteristic of osteomas.

		The newly formed, mature bone is arranged in layers, suggesting periodic growth. A concentric, lamellar bony organisation gives rise to the classic 'onion-skin' histologic appearance.
55	J	Osteoma ➢ Osteoma is the most common benign tumour of the temporal bone. It tends to be unilateral pedunculated mass that is more common in males. It originates from the tympanosquamous or tympanomastoid suture lines at the bony-cartilaginous junction. ➢ Histology reveals well-formed lamellae with multiple fibrovascular channels throughout the interlamellar spaces. ➢ Osteomas manifest with similar symptoms as exostoses including conductive hearing loss, otorrhea, otalgia, otitis externa and cholesteatoma. Unusual presentations of osteoma include unilateral headache and as an EAC polyp. ➢ On CT scan findings of exostoses appear as broad based lesion with no deep extension, while an osteoma is seen as a well-demarcated, hyper-

		dense attenuating outgrowth tumor. Both coronal and axial scans are helpful in demonstrating the exact dimensions and complications, such as canal cholesteatoma developing medial to osteoma and exostosis.
56	H	Keratosis Obturans ➢ This condition may present with a conductive hearing loss due to the accumulation of large plugs of desquamated keratin in the ear canal. ➢ The condition is thought to arise due to altered migration of squamous epithelium from ear canal. ➢ Keratosis of the tympanic membrane alone has been reported and may presents as tinnitus. ➢ The accumulation of sheets of keratin in the canal leads to circumferential erosion of the canal and automastoidectomy. The debris may become infected and mimic standard otitis externa. The keratin plug seen in keratosis obturans appears like a geometrically patterned keratin plug within the lumen of expanded ear canal. These keratin squames are shed from the complete circumference of the deep ear canal forming a lamina. It appears like

		onion skin. ➢ Management includes removal of keratin under general anaesthetic, canaloplasty for recurrent cases and mastoidectomy for cases with primary external canal cholesteatoma.
57	E	External auditory canal cholesteatoma ➢ This condition can occur spontaneously or post operatively. Its aetiology is unclear but thought to occur after entrapment of squamous epithelium during the healing process. ➢ It presents with unilateral discharge and chronic dull pain as the localised bone posteroinferiorly is eroded. ➢ A cholesteatoma is a cystic structure lined by keratinising stratified squamous epithelium with associated periostitis and bone erosion, which is most commonly found in the middle ear cavity. ➢ Middle ear cholesteatomas may be congenital or acquired, but approximately 98% are acquired. ➢ The incidence of EACC is 0.1–0.5% of all otologic patients. ➢ Differential diagnoses, including neoplasms of the EAC, keratosis

		obturans, postinflammatory medial canal fibrosis, and necrotising (malignant) otitis externa. ➢ Keratosis obturans is often bilateral, occurs in younger population and rarely presents with discharge. EACC is thought to occur either spontaneously, due to poor keratin migration, or secondary after ear surgery. ➢ Spontaneous cases can be managed with regular suction clearance as long as the mastoid is not invaded. Post surgical cases almost always require surgery. A modified radical mastoidectomy is recommended if the mastoid is invaded.
58	I	Necrotising otitis externa ➢ This is an infectious process in an immunocompromised or diabetic patient. In diabetics the pH of the ear canal is higher and polymorphonuclear cell dysfunction, which provides healthy environment for Pseudomonas aeruginosa to grow in, which is the commonest pathogen. This bacterium does not normally live in the external ear canal. ➢ The infection invades ear cartilage

		and then spreads to the temporal bone via the fissures of Santorini. This gives rise to granulation tissue at the bony cartilaginous interface. Facial nerve paralysis is the most common cranial nerve pathology (75%) and confers a worse prognosis compared to no cranial nerve involvement. ➢ CT scan with contrast can be helpful in diagnosing and staging the disease but Gallium-67 scan is useful for monitoring therapy. Mortality is between 20–54%. ➢ Pain is a good marker of disease state and long term antibiotics are the mainstay of treatment. Otitis that is not controlled with antibiotics may benefit from surgical debridement of necrotic bone.
59	I	Superficial spreading malignant melanoma ➢ With regard to malignant melanoma exposure to sunlight is a major aetiological factor. Malignant transformation in a mole should be suspected if there are changes in size, shape or colour. ➢ Other changes that are not as significant include inflammation, crusting/bleeding, itching and diameter a 6 mm or more.

- Familial malignant melanoma accounts for 8–12% of all melanomas. They tend to occur at a younger age. Around 3–5% of patients who have been diagnosed with melanoma go on to develop a second primary.
- Histopathological types of melanoma are as follows:
    - Superficial spreading melanoma. This is the most common form of melanoma, accounting for 70% of all cutaneous melanomas. The peak incidence is in the fifth decade of life. The common site in men is the back and in women the legs.
    - Lentigo maligna melanoma. This is the most benign form of melanoma being slow growing, it accounts for 10–15% of all cutaneous melanomas.
    - Nodular melanoma are the most malignant type of malignant melanoma, they are twice as common in men. Clinically these lesions develop quickly.
    - Acral lentiginous melanoma is

		observed on the palms, soles, under the nails and in the oral mucosa. It occurs on non hair-bearing surfaces of the body which may or may not be exposed to sunlight. It is also found on mucous membranes. Unlike other forms of melanoma, acral lentiginous melanoma does not appear to be linked to sun exposure.
60	E	Keratoacanthoma ➢ This condition is more common in males with a ratio of 2:1 and in the 7th decade of life. ➢ Keratoacanthoma is a rapidly growing epidermal tumour that bares the hallmarks of squamous cell carcinoma both clinically and histologically. It is believed to arise from pilosebaceous glands. ➢ There is limited evidence that keratoacanthoma has malignant potential but it may mimic histological features of squamous cell carcinoma. In fact, strong arguments support classifying keratoacanthoma as a variant of invasive SCC as it shares similar characteristic to SCC

		and Bowen's disease (SCC in situ). It is differentiated from SCC with its rapid growth to 1–2cm in a few weeks and spontaneous resolution leaving a scar after a few months. ➢ Physical examination shows a reddish papule with a keratin filled crater. ➢ Various aetiological agents have been implicated including trauma, viral infection, sun exposure, and long term exposure to tar. ➢ Surgical excision is often not indicated, especially on the nose where reconstruction is surgically challenging.
61	B	Basal cell carcinomas ➢ Basal cell carcinomas are the most common cancers in human but account for only 0.1% of all cancer related mortality. ➢ These are slow-growing, locally invasive malignant epidermal skin tumours that originate from the basal layer of the epidermis. Invasion into the dermis is common but spread elsewhere is rare. ➢ They predominantly affect Caucasians and are rare in dark skinned races. 70% of BCCs occur on the face. It is more common at points of

		embryological fusion. ➢ The skin changes caused by this skin cancer depend on the type of basal cell carcinoma involved. The most common appearance is of a raised pink or pearly white bump that may have a translucent, rolled, pearly edge and telangiectasias. ➢ Differential includes squamous cell carcinoma and melanoma. ➢ Resection margins and treatment is different for all 3. Therefore a biopsy of the lesion is advisable. Treatment can by topical chemotherapy such as imiquimod or fluorouracil, cryotherapy or surgery. Surgery should take 3–4 mm of health tissue to ensure clearance.
62	F	Papilloma. ➢ Papilloma refers to a benign epithelial tumour growing exophytically in finger-like fronds. In this context papilla refers to the projection created by the tumor, not a tumor on an already existing papilla (such as the nipple). When used without context, it frequently refers to infections caused by human papillomavirus (HPV), such as warts. ➢ There are, however, a number of

			other conditions that cause papilloma and in many cases there is no known cause. A squamous cell papilloma is a generally benign papilloma that arises from the stratified squamous epithelium of the skin, lip, oral cavity, tongue, pharynx, larynx, esophagus, cervix, vagina or anal canal. ➢ Squamous cell papillomas are a result of infection with human papillomavirus (HPV). Nasal papillomas are very common wart-like growths arising from the nasal vestibule. They tend to cause irritation or be cosmetically undesirable. They will bleed if traumatised. ➢ Treatment is by excision under local anaesthesia. ➢ Squamous cell papilloma of the mouth or throat is generally diagnosed in people between the ages of 30–50, and is normally found on the inside of the cheek, on the tongue, or inside of lips. Oral papillomas are usually painless, and not treated unless they interfere with eating or are causing pain. They do not generally mutate to cancerous

		growths, nor do they normally grow or spread. Oral papillomas are most usually a result of the infection with types HPV-6 and HPV-11. ➢ Conjunctival squamous cell papilloma are normally found in children or young adults, a common cause of conjunctival squamous cell papilloma is during childbirth, when the mother passes the virus to her child.
63	A	Aspirin ➢ She most likely would have taken aspirin which is easily available. ➢ Salicylates can cause a reversible hearing loss. Apart from that it also causes tinnitus. The incidence rate is less than 1%. Elderly patients are at a significantly high risk of salicylate toxicity even at lower salicylate doses. Tinnitus also occurs with salicylates with the usual frequency of tinnitus being in the 7–9 k Hz range. Tinnitus may be used as an initial sign of salicylate ototoxicity and may be used as a baseline in patients with normal initial hearing. It is believed that the mechanism of salicylate ototoxicity is related to reversible biochemical or metabolic changes in the cochlear rather than

		any permanent morphologic abnormality. ➢ Please note that quinine also causes significant tinnitus. ➢ Acute salicylate poisoning causes hyperventilation, respiratory alkalosis and metabolic acidosis. Since all the symptoms are reversible, a patient who is complaining of aspirin-induced tinnitus should be reassured that he or she will get better in 24–48 hours.
64	D	Gentamicin ➢ Ototoxicity is reduced cochleovestibular function as a result of interaction of chemicals. There are a great number of ototoxic substances but only a few in common therapeutic uses. ➢ The two most commonly described ototoxic agents are platinum-based chemotherapeutic agents and aminoglycoside antibiotic. The patient in the clinical scenario most likely would have received intravenous gentamicin (an aminoglycoside) for his bladder infection. ➢ The incidence of ototoxicity after aminoglycoside is dose dependent and ranges from 2–45% after intake

		for four consecutive days. Patients typically present with bilateral high frequency hearing loss that may be accompanied by peripheral vestibular hypofunction. ➢ The mechanism of aminoglycoside ototoxicity appears to involve both apoptotic pathways as well as formation of free radicals. Some are predominantly cochleotoxic (neomycin, amikacin, tobramycin, kanamycin) whilst others are preferentially vestibulotoxic (gentamicin and streptomycin). ➢ Some individuals have an unusual susceptibility to gentamicin or streptomycin ototoxicity related to a mutation of mitochondrial RNA. This susceptibility is passed on genetically through the mother and occurs in as many as 17% of individuals with hearing loss after aminoglycoside exposure. ➢ Heat shock proteins (Hsp) may play a protective role in aminoglycoside toxicity. ➢ Other ototoxic drugs are loop diuretics, organophosphates and quinine.

65	H	Propanolol ➢ Beta blockers can cause a mixed deafness. The conductive element is caused by a middle ear effusion but the pathogenesis of the effusion and the cochleotoxicity has not been elucidated. The effects are generally reversible. Propranolol is a fat soluble beta blocker which crosses the blood brain barrier and can be used for tremor. However, it also causes severe nightmares and use should be judicious. ➢ When taking a history of someone with hearing loss it is vital to get a good drug history. This will help elucidate reversible causes which can be corrected. It is also to note that although some medications cause irreversible hearing loss, continuing on them can precipitate a further deterioration in hearing. ➢ Conductive hearing losses can be corrected surgically if necessary and sensorineural causes can be augmented with hearing aids. Cochlear implantation is the final step for profound bilateral sensory hearing loss.

66	B	Laryngotracheal injury ➢ Laryngotracheal injuries are relatively uncommon with an estimated incidence of 1% of all trauma cases. They may be associated with fractures of the facial skeleton. ➢ Their symptoms are variable ranging from obvious airway obstruction to minor or nonexistent. ➢ Early diagnosis and proper initial management may sometimes be difficult or delayed. ➢ Subcutaneous emphysema is the chief clinical sign. ➢ Fibreoptic endoscopy is the most important and informative diagnostic examination. Radiographic evaluation by CT scan provides additional information about the extent of the injury and the indication for surgery. ➢ Because of airway compromise from swelling of tissue such as the laryngeal mucosa and tongue base, one should have a low threshold for tracheostomy. In penetrating neck injury with progressive dyspnoea it is important to perform a surgical exploration.
67	F	Pinna haematoma ➢ Pinna haematoma or subchondral

		haematoma of the ear usually results from some sort of shearing injury. Nutrition to all cartilage in the body comes from the perichondrium. Blood vessels are present in the perichondrial plane and a shearing force causes them to tear and bleed into the subperichondrial plane. This prevents nutrition from the perichondrium getting to the cartilage, leading to eventual cartilage necrosis and cauliflowering of the ear. ➢ For this reason the condition should be dealt with promptly and effectively. This may require a general anaesthesia to ensure complete drainage and apposition of the perichondrial layer to the cartilage with sutures over a splint.
68	A	T1N0 ➢ TNM stages of nasopharyngeal cancer describes: the size of a pr mary tumour (T): whether the cancer has spread to the lymph nodes (N) and whether the cancer has spread to a different part of the body (M). ➢ There are four main stages in this system – stages 1–4. A very early stage cancer is sometimes referred to

		as stage 0 or carcinoma in situ. ➢ The grade of a cancer tells you how much the cancer cells look like normal cells. If you have a low grade cancer, the cancer cells look very much like normal nasopharyngeal cells. High grade means they look very abnormal and very unlike normal nasopharyngeal cells. High grade cancers are likely to be faster growing and are more likely to spread. But in nasopharyngeal cancer, high grade cancers can respond particularly well to treatment with radiotherapy. ➢ There are different ways of staging cancers. The two main ways are the TNM system and number system. They are used together to give doctor a description of the cancer.
69	F	T2 N1
70	H	Temporal arteritis ➢ Also called Giant-cell arteritis (GCA) is a chronic vascular disease of unknown origin. It is characterised by granulomatous inflammation in the wall of medium-size and large arteries. It is more common in females than males by a ratio of 3:1. The mean age of onset is about 70 years. ➢ Symptoms include; bruits, fever,

		headache, tenderness and sensitivity on the scalp, jaw claudication, tongue claudication, reduced visual acuity, acute visual loss, diplopia and acute tinnitus. ➢ Erythrocyte sedimentation rate, an inflammatory marker is useful it is usually >60 mm/hour (normal 10–40 mm/hour), but may be normal in approximately 20% of cases. Other screening includes C-reactive protein and platelets may also be elevated. A risk of this disease is blindness and so early and long term use of steroids is recommended.
71	D	Migraine ➢ This is a common disabling primary headache disorder. It is the most common cause of recurrent disabling headache. Migraine is a syndrome which is characterised by periodic headaches with complete resolution between attacks. Attacks may be composed of the following stages: a prodrome, aura, headache and resolution. The frequency of attacks is variable from several per week to several per lifetime. ➢ A prodrome is a vague change in mood or appetite, and aura however,

		is a clear neurological symptom such as a visual disturbance or motor or sensory disturbance. Underlying mechanisms are thought to be related to vasospasms and neurotransmitter imbalance. ➢ Treatment has focused on removing triggering factors, basic analgesia and serotonin analogues. The neurological deficit can occur in any region and patients can have severe vertigo as a presenting feature.
72	G	Young's syndrome ➢ This is the triad of bronchiectasis, rhinosinusitis and reduced fertility. The syndrome was named after Donald Young, the urologist who first made observations of the clinical signs of the syndrome in 1972. ➢ Ciliary activity and lung function is normal but the mucus is abnormally viscus. Reduced fertility is due to functional obstruction of sperm transport down the genital tract at the level of the caput epididymis where the sperm are found in viscous, lipid-rich fluid.
73	C	Cystic Fibrosis ➢ This is one of the UK's most common

			life-threatening inherited diseases. It is a chronic, multisystem disorder characterised by recurrent endo-bronchial infections, progressive obstructive pulmonary disease and pancreatic insufficiency with intestinal malabsorption. ➢ The frequency of nasal polyposis in sinonasal disease related to CF is quite variable and is believed to be in the range of 6–67% of patients. It is an autosomal recessive condition with a defect on the CFTR gene that codes for chloride channels causing a very salty sweat. This forms the basis of the most commonly used diagnostic test. ➢ It can present in infancy with meconium ileus or in early childhood with failure to thrive. This is related to poor nutritional intake due to pancreatic insuffiency, as well as lung complications. Lung and sinus problems occur due to accumulation of thick mucous which is difficult to clear. This leads to poor mucociliary flow and eventual blockage with ensuing inflammation. Eventually there is change in the underlying anatomy, such as bronchiectasis in

		the lung and polyposis in the sinuses. ➢ One should consider this condition in a young child who presents with nasal polyposis. The use of viral vectors to transpose the defective gene is currently being tested, but until then treatment is expectant.
74	D	Kartagener's syndrome ➢ This is an autosomal recessive condition that results from primary ciliary dyskinesia. Incidence is 1 in 32,000 births. ➢ This is the combination of bronchiectasis, sinusitis and dextrocardia. ➢ Ciliated epithelium covers most areas of the upper respiratory tract, including the nasal mucosa, paranasal sinuses, middle ear, eustachian tube, and pharynx. The lower respiratory tract contains ciliated epithelium from the trachea to the respiratory bronchioles. Each ciliated cell gives rise to approximately 200 cilia that vary in length from 5–6 μm and decrease in size as the airway becomes smaller. ➢ Sinus imaging typically demonstrate mucosal thickening, opacified sinus cavities, and hypoplastic frontal

		sinuses.
75	J	Laryngomalacia ➢ The 3-month-old has laryngomalacia which can present soon after birth. It is the most common cause of stridor in infants. The shortened aryepiglottic folds cause the epiglottis to be furled in on itself. This is the well known 'omega shaped' epiglottis. ➢ A classification system has been proposed. In type 1 laryngomalacia, the aryepiglottic folds are tightened or foreshortened. Type 2 is marked by redundant soft tissue in any area of the supraglottic region. Type 3 is associated with other disorders, such as neuromuscular disease and gastroesophageal reflux. ➢ Laryngomalacia is normally a self-limiting condition, but occasionally the stridor becomes severe with signs of respiratory distress and distressed feeding. ➢ If growth is affected surgery is recommended. Surgery can take the form of a tracheostomy in the severest forms but on the whole involves an aryepiglottoplasty. Aryepiglottoplasty involves division or

		excision of the aryepiglottic folds, with occasional excision of the cuneiform cartilage and attaching the epiglottis to the tongue base with laser and or stitches.
76	A	Acute epiglottitis ➢ The 4-year-old is suffering from acute epiglottitis; which is a life-threatening medical emergency. The priority is to secure the child's airway causing minimal distress. This requires effective multidisciplinary input including a senior anaesthetist, paediatrician and ENT surgeon. The child should be transferred to an anaesthetic room with a view to endotracheal intubation. Intravenous antibiotics and steroids are commenced afterwards. ➢ Haemophilus influenzae type B is the most common causative organism, though the introduction of vaccination has resulted in a significant reduction in incidence of acute epiglottitis. Other causes include Streptococcus pneumoniae, varicella-zoster, herpes simplex virus type 1 and Staphylococcus aureus. ➢ During an acute attack it is extremely painful to swallow and due to

		infection there are increased secretions. The child is deliberately holding these secretions in the oropharynx. ➢ Any overstimulation with needles, examinations or intubation attempts can lead to sudden rapid aspiration of secretions and respiratory arrest. This is the reason that the child should be kept in a calm soothing environment whilst senior members of the multidisciplinary team are convened. It's only in theatre that anything should be attempted in case of need to perform an urgent tracheostomy.
77	I	Laryngeal papillomatosis ➢ The 7-year-old girl has laryngeal papillomatosis, which is characterised by benign wart-like lesions that can affect any part of the respiratory tract. The causative organisms are human papillomavirus types 6 and 11. Maternal transmission by mothers affected with genital warts through vaginal birth is believed to be the main source of infection. ➢ In babies and small children the symptoms include a weak cry, trouble swallowing, noisy breathing, and chronic cough. Dysphonia and stridor

		may be present in advanced cases. ➢ Treatment requires laser excision of differing intervals. Tracheostomy is not recommended because of the risk of implantation of papilloma into trachea and bronchi. ➢ Papillomata in the trachea have a small risk of malignant transformation due to squamous metaplasia, whereas laryngeal papillomatosis have no risk of malignancy. Treatment never removes all the virus latent in the mucosa. Therefore, treatment should not be aggressive stripping of the larynx but rather driven towards symptom relief.
78	H	Foreign body. ➢ The 2-year-old has a typical presentation an inhaled foreign body. The presentation is dependent on its size and the nature of the foreign body; organic or inorganic, benign or caustic. ➢ A small inorganic foreign body may present with a brief episode of choking, cyanosis and little else. Occasionally a chest X-ray may be helpful in identifying the foreign body. There may be occlusion of a

		bronchus with subsequent collapse of a lobe causing respiratory distress. ➢ Larger foreign bodies may result in occlusion of the airway at the level of the larynx with potential laryngospasm and death. ➢ Organic foreign bodies (e.g. a nut) can cause marked inflammation in the lower airways due to the irritation the mucosa. Removal via a bronchoscope can be difficult as organic material tends to fragment. The key to success is team approach with suitable equipment such as a ventilating bronchoscope and optical forceps.
79	B	Cholesteatoma. ➢ A cholesteatoma is an expansive destructive growth consisting of keratinising squamous epithelium in the middle ear and/or mastoid process. Symptoms depend on the activity of the disease and can be due to the lesion itself or its complications. ➢ Congenital cholesteatomas arise as a consequence of squamous epithelium trapped within the temporal bone during embryogenesis. ➢ Primary acquired cholesteatomas

			arise as the result of tympanic membrane retraction. The classic primary acquired cholesteatoma develops from progressively deeper medial retraction of the pars flaccida into the epitympanum. A second type of primary acquired cholesteatomas arises when the posterior quadrant of the tympanic membrane is retracted into the posterior middle ear. The drum initially adheres to the long process of the incus. As retraction continues medially and posteriorly, squamous epithelium envelops the superstructure of the stapes and retracts into the sinus tympani. ➢ Secondary acquired cholesteatomas occur as a direct consequence of some type of injury to the tympanic membrane. ➢ Cholesteatoma is a surgical disease and if possible is best treated with tympanomastoid surgery. It must be remembered that the disease process is microscopic and complete clearance can never be assured hence the need for a second look operation if a closed cavity approach is used. ➢ A diffusion weighted MRI scan regime is proving of some use in following up

		operated patients. ➢ Anatomically the facial recess tends to be the site of common recurrence because it's poor accessibility.
80	A	Acoustic neuroma ➢ An acoustic neuroma is a benign, slow growing neoplasm of the vestibulocochlear nerve cells of the eighth cranial nerve. These tumours comprise around 6% of all intracranial tumors. The lesions are usually located in the internal auditory canal (intracanalicular) or the cerebellopontine angle (intracranial) causing compression of the vestibular nerve and resulting eventually in deafness. Continued growth of the neuroma may compress the brain stem and cause related symptoms. ➢ The main considerations for treatment include age and co-morbid status of patient, size of tumour, location and patient preference and hearing loss. ➢ Treatment modalities include conservative repeat scanning, surgical excision (translabyrinthine and retrosigmoid approaches) and gamma knife radiotherapy. Young patients warrant tumour destruction

		as the neuroma will likely continue to grow over their life and proof more difficult to treat. Tumours less than 1cm are normally serially scanned, whereas those over 2cm normally require treatment.
81	E	Otitis externa ➢ Otitis externa is a diffuse inflammation of the skin lining the external auditory meatus. Causative agents of infective otitis externa include: ➢ Infection: Bacterial (90%) -especially staphylococcus. Fungal (10%) -candida, aspergillus ➢ Allergy -eczema; contact allergy to cosmetics, shampoos ➢ Trauma -e.g. cotton bud ➢ Otitis externa is more prevalent in people with narrowed or tortuous canal ear canals. Other precipitants include moisture, foreign objects in the ear canal (hearing aids etc.) and chronic skin diseases (e.g. Psoriasis). ➢ Treatment should include taking swabs for microbiology, microsuction debridement and topical acidifying agents and antibiotics. Exacerbating factors should be addressed for

		recurrent conditions. ➢ Complications of untreated disease include spread to temporal bone (malignant otitis externa) and subsequent cranial nerve palsies (Gradenigo's syndrome).
82	D	Impacted wax ➢ The lady in the Jacuzzi may have submerged her head causing water to enter the ear canal. This caused expansion of the wax plug which may have been present for a long time. ➢ Wax or cerumen is composed of secretions and sloughed epithelial cells and hair from the external auditory canal. It protects the skin in the canal and is naturally extruded. However, cerumen may accumulate and occlude the canal of one or both ears, causing discomfort, hearing loss, tinnitus, dizziness, and cough. ➢ Large amounts of wax in the canal have little impact, yet smaller quantities on the tympanic membrane can precipitate significant clinical symptoms. ➢ Treatment involves removal of wax. This can be done by wax softening drops (olive oil, sodium hydrogen bicarbonate) which makes natural

		migration of wax easier. ➢ Another option includes syringing water into the canal which will bypass the wax, hit the drum and on return push the wax out of the ear. However, this can traumatise the canal or the drum and in some cases has precipitated a tympanic membrane perforation. ➢ Alternatively the use of microscope with fine suction can remove wax under direct visualisation, but requires equipment and expertise.
83	I	Tracheal web ➢ A tracheal web consists of a thin layer of tissue draped across the tracheal lumen. While the thickness of the web may vary, no deformity or abnormality of the underlying cartilage framework exists. The web is not complete; the degree of ventilatory symptoms present is directly related to the size of the remaining tracheal lumen. ➢ Treatment consists of rupturing the web. This may be accomplished via steroid injection, balloon dilatation and laser division to widen the lumen. ➢ Congenital tracheal malformations

			may be intrinsic to the trachea per se or represent external forces compressing the airway. Although strictly speaking congenital tracheal malformations are present at birth, at times they may not cause symptoms until far later in life. ➢ The primary presenting symptom is most commonly biphasic stridor, with a considerably prolonged expiratory phase. Nevertheless, other airway-related symptoms (e.g. wheezing, cough, pneumonia, croup) may be present as well. ➢ A history of frequent neck hyperextension is common as the child tries to maximally open the airway. ➢ Many tests are available to assist in the workup of congenital tracheal malformations. Barium swallow studies may reveal extrinsic esophageal compression. In a child with dysphagia, a dynamic fluoroscopic study may be considered. CT scanning of the neck and chest provides additional data, while MRI together with magnetic resonance angiography (MRA) can provide detailed vascular information

		and may obviate the need for conventional contrast angiography. However, the criterion standard diagnostic modality is still direct laryngoscopy with rigid bronchoscopy and possible rigid esophagoscopy.
84	J	Tracheomalacia ➢ In tracheomalacia, the supporting structure of the trachea (anterior cartilage) is too floppy, resulting from weakness of the tracheal walls. In addition, the posterior or membranous portion of the trachea (trachealis muscle), which does not add support to the trachea, may be wider than normal. ➢ Patients exhibit an expiratory stridor, which may resemble wheezing. During heavy breathing, the membranous posterior wall advances anteriorly, where it may approach or even touch the cartilaginous anterior tracheal wall, thus markedly reducing the airway lumen. ➢ Symptoms of tracheomalacia are generally self-limiting because adequate growth in the diameter of the trachea eliminates symptoms by the time the patient is aged 2 years. ➢ Diagnosis is difficult due to as rigid

		bronchoscopy under general anaesthetic will stent open the airway and no collapse will be seen. Flexible bronchoscopy and lung flow volume loops are required. ➢ For severe cases, tracheotomy, continuous positive airway pressure (CPAP), or both may be necessary until the tracheomalacia is outgrown.
85	A	Bat/prominent ears ➢ Prominent ears are the butt of teasing, unpleasantness and bullying. This can carry on into areas that give rise to protruding ears but only one may be present. There are three anatomical regions; antihelix, large conchal bowl and protruding lobule which could lead to this condition and should be assessed during consultation. ➢ Treatment options include camouflaging technique and otoplasty surgery. There are various techniques, few of which are Furnas conchomastoid suture and Mustarde suturing method. Large conchal bowl may be partially excised or stitched. Protruding lobule requires sectioning of the cauda helicis. Surgery can be carried out from the age of 5: the ear

		is well formed by this stage and teasing has not usually started before this. ➢ A special dressing is round the head to hold it all in place. After going home, it is very important to leave the bandage alone: if it comes off, it is best re-applied at the Hospital. The bandage stays on for about 8 days when it is removed at the Hospital. There is some bruising and swelling at this stage which settles quickly. The bandage is worn at home at night for a further 3 applied to each ear to keep the new shape and a bandage, held with tape, is then wound weeks. The stitches behind the ear take about 4 weeks to fall out. Contact sports should be avoided during this time. ➢ Exact symmetry of the ears is not guaranteed (most people's ears are a bit different from each other). Very occasionally, the initial result requires slight alteration and, if required, this would normally be done after about 6 months.
86	G	Submucous cleft ➢ A submucous cleft of the soft palate is characterised by a midline

		deficiency or lack of muscular tissue and incorrect positioning of the muscles. A submucous cleft of the hard palate is defined as a bony defect in the midline or centre of the bony palate. Often a submucous cleft palate is associated with a bifid or cleft uvula. ➢ In patients requiring adenoidectomy a bifid uvula and submucous cleft of the soft palate should always be examined for. In this subset of patients an andenoidectomy can lead to nasal regurgitation of food and therefore the procedure should be avoided. ➢ A cleft palate is normally diagnosed at birth during the neonatal screen and presents with nasal aspiration during feeding. Surgical correction should be always be attempted. There is no need to surgically correct a submucous cleft.
87	A	Cogan's syndrome ➢ Cogan syndrome is a condition characterized by recurrent inflammation of the cornea and often fever, fatigue, and weight loss, episodes of dizziness, and hearing loss. It is associated with deafness or

<table>
<tr>
<td></td>
<td></td>
<td></td>
<td>blindness if untreated.
➢ Cogan's syndrome is most probably an autoimmune disease. Autoantibodies may be found in the blood of some patients, and these antibodies have been shown to attack inner ear tissue. The condition may also be associated with vasculitis in other areas of the body that can cause major organ damage in 15% of those afflicted or, in a small number of cases, even death.
➢ Oral corticosteroids may be necessary to reduce the inflammatory response. When large amounts of steroids are required or if the disease is severe and is not responding to steroid therapy, other immunosuppressive medications such as methotrexate (Rheumatrex), cyclophosphamide (Cytoxan, Neosar), cyclosporine (Neoral, Sandimmune) or azathioprine (Imuran) may be needed. In some cases, combinations of these medicines are prescribed.
➢ Occasionally, if the disease has damaged blood vessels, cochlear implantation may need to be done to correct the problem. Studies have shown it to produce significant</td>
</tr>
</table>

		improvement in hearing loss in some patients.

88	H	Systemic lupus erythematosus
		➢ Systemic lupus erythematosus is a multiorgan system autoimmune disease with numerous immunological and clinical manifestations. It is characterised by an auto-antibody response to nuclear and cytoplasmic antigens. The disease mainly involves the skin, joints, kidneys, blood cells, and nervous system.
		➢ Classification Criteria for the Diagnosis of Systemic Lupus Erythematosus
		  ➢ Malar rash: Fixed erythema, flat or raised, over the malar eminences
		  ➢ Discoid rash: Erythematous circular raised patches with adherent keratotic scaling and follicular plugging; atrophic scarring may occur
		  ➢ Photosensitivity: Exposure to ultraviolet light causes rash
		  ➢ Oral ulcers: Includes oral and nasopharyngeal ulcers, observed by physician
		  ➢ Arthritis: Nonerosive arthritis of

		two or more peripheral joints, with tenderness, swelling, or effusion ➢ Serositis: Pleuritis or pericarditis documented by ECG or rub or evidence of effusion ➢ Renal disorder: Proteinuria >0.5 g/d or 3+, or cellular casts ➢ Neurologic disorder: Seizures or psychosis without other causes ➢ Hematologic disorder: Haemolytic anemia or leucopenia (<4000/L) or lymphopenia (<1500/L) or thrombocytopenia (<100,000/L) in the absence of offending drugs ➢ Immunologic disorder: Anti-dsDNA, anti-Sm, and/or anti-phospholipid Antinuclear antibodies.
89	F	Sjögren's syndrome ➢ Primary Sjögren's syndrome is the association of keratoconjunctivitis sicca and/or xerostomia, with rheumatoid arthritis or other connective tissue disorder. ➢ No single test exists for diagnosis. SS-A (or Ro) and SS-B (or La) are the marker antibodies for Sjögren's. Seventy per cent of Sjögren's patients

		are positive for SS-A and 40% are positive for SS-B (these may also found in lupus patients). Other tests include ANA (Anti-Nuclear Antibody). ANAs are a group of antibodies that react against normal components of a cell nucleus. About 70% of Sjögren's patients have a positive ANA test result. ➢ Salivary gland biopsy shows sialadenitis. ➢ Involvement of other secretory glands is common causing dyspareunia, dry skin, dysphagia, otitis media and pulmonary infection. ➢ Other features include dental caries, attacks of monilial stomatitis, neuropathy, hepatosplenomegaly and renal involvement. Associations include renal tubular acidosis, adverse drug reactions and lymphoma. ➢ Secondary Sjögren's occurs in about 50% of cases of rheumatoid arthritis.
90	C	Leprosy ➢ Leprosy (Hansen's disease) is a chronic mycobacterial disease caused by Mycobacteria Leprae, an acid-fast bacillus. Skin lesions are the primary external sign, whilst lepromatous

		deposits on nerves can lead to other deformities (such as saddle nose deformity) because of loss of sensation. ➢ The disease can be subclassified into two entities depending on a patient's immune response to the disease. Those who exhibit a strong response have fewer skin lesions and asymmetrical neuropathy. Whereas those who have minimal response to the disease have large number of skin lesions and symmetrical neuropathy. ➢ Neuropathies of facial and greater auricular nerve have all been detailed in the past. The condition is more common in men compared to women with a ratio of 1.5:1. ➢ Multidrug treatment with dapsone and rifampicin has led to a drop in worldwide incidence but the WHO drive to eradicate the disease by 2000 failed.
91	E	Surgery can proceed ➢ Informed consent is bound by ethical and legal frameworks, and the processes for obtaining it must be independently scrutinised and approved. ➢ For any consent to be legally valid,

		regardless of the age of the patient, three principles have to be met: (i) competence (ii) voluntariness of the decision and (iii) the information on which the patient has to base his or her decision. ➢ The Mental Health act is not as far reaching as allowing for treatment of conditions other than the mental disorder. The surgeon may proceed in the patient's best interest. However, it is good clinical practice to obtain a second surgical opinion confirming the need for intervention as well as involving the relatives.
92	A	Make patient ward of court ➢ The Jehovah Witness question raises a number of issues. A surgeon could respect the patients wishes, most however would proceed by applying to make the child a ward of court. The consent process is vital to surgery. It ensures the patient has fully understood the repercussions of surgery, with the chance of success and risk of complications ➢ Consent form 1 is a basic adult consent form. Consent form 2 is for paediatric patients. Parents or guardians must sign this form on

		behalf of the child. Consent form 3 is patient agreement to investigation or treatrment where consciousness is not impaired. Consent form 4 is for patients who are unable to consent and is completed by healthcare professionals detailing the reason the procedure was performed.
93	E	Surgery can proceed ➢ The surgery for the lady is required for preservation of life and can be performed despite the patient's inability to give consent. The Mental Capacity Act 2005 and in Scotland: The Adults with Incapacity Act 2000 says that competent individuals over 18 (over 16 in Scotland) can appoint someone to make decisions about medical treatment on their behalf if they become unable to do so (Lasting Power of Attorney). If no such power of attorney has been executed then no one can consent to or refuse treatment on behalf of an adult. Advance refusals (living wills) are normally legally binding.
94	D	Bone anchored hearing aid (on a soft band) ➢ This baby has Treacher–collins syndrome. He can wear a soft band bone conduction hearing aid until he

is suitable for surgery.

- The bone-anchored hearing aid (BAHA) is an alternative to traditional bone conductor hearing aids and overcomes the problems with poor sound quality, high battery consumption, poor aesthetics and insecure positioning of the device. Whereas conventional bone conductors work transcutaneously, losing some sound energy through the soft tissues, BAHA works percutaneously resulting in better sound quality.
- A small titanium fixture is implanted into the skull behind the ear where it osseointegrates with the living bone. An abutment is attached to the fixture and the processor is clipped on and can be worn or taken off at any time. The newer BAHA (Sophono) utilizes implanted magnets to hold the processor in place. The surgical procedure is relatively minor and can be performed under local or general anaesthesia.
- Bone anchored hearing aids are currently being used in patients with conductive or mixed hearing losses that are not surgically rectifiable or

		who are unable to tolerate traditional hearing device because of conditions such as chronic otitis external, atresia, stenosis, mastoiditis or iatrogenic obliteration of the external auditory canal. ➢ Bilateral congenital canal atresia remains the absolute indication. ➢ Patient selection is vital and all patients should undergo a trial period of wearing a bone conduction aid supported with a headband. Though the surgical procedure is relatively straightforward, complications may result with failure of the graft or implant, as a result of infection. ➢ The use of bone anchored hearing has been approved for the treatment of single sided deafness or unilateral sensorineural deafness. This could be idiopathic, traumatic or post surgical. The device passes bone-conducted sound vibration from the temporal bone behind the dead ear over the skull to the other side where it stimulates the cochlea of the good ear. This restores the sensation of hearing from the deaf side, and, after a period of adaptation, some patients may develop the capacity for

		localisation of sound in space and this ultimately improves their quality of life.
95	H	Brainstem implant ➢ The abscent cochlea means that cochlear implants are totally unsuitable as there is no anatomical structure to implant. The auditory brainstem implant has been developed in an endeavour to address those who dont have functioning coclear nerves. The idea is to stimulate directly the auditory brainstem. ➢ The implant consists of a platinium electrode array connected to an implant receiver/stimulator package. The position of the electrode array is checked electrophysiologically at the time of surgery. Most implanted patients use temporal cues as it helps to improve lip-reading skills. Nearly all patients experience non-auditory sensations, which can be reduced by adjustments to the pattern and frequency of the electrode stimulation. With adequate training, the performance of brainstem implanted patients can rival those with cochlear implant.

		➢ However, the operation is a major neurosurgical procedure and carries all the complications associated with intracranial operations.
96	C	Bilateral cochlear implants ➢ NICE guidelines recommend early bilateral cochlear implants for hearing loss following meningitis because of the cochlear ossification sequelae. Meningitis causes damage to the cochlear hair cells. Cochlear implants bypass this problem by directly stimulating the spiral ganglion cells of the auditory nerve. ➢ A cochlear implant consists of two components: an external processor and a surgically implanted internal electrode coil. A small external microphone converts signal into electrical energy. This is conveyed to an external speech processor. Here the information is coded and transmitted to an implanted receiver/stimulator percutaneously via a coil transmitter which is held in position by magnetic attraction to the implant. The signal is decoded by the receiver and then forwarded to the stimulator electrode array placed surgically in the scala tympani of the

			cochlea. ➢ The current theory is that the implanted electrodes directly stimulate the spiral ganglion cells of the cochlear nerve. Patients experience considerable benefits. When wearing the external processor, they are able to hear speech and music and to use the telephone. ➢ The selection criteria for cochlear implants are constantly evolving and changing with the advancements in implant technology. The process of selecting appropriate individuals for implantation usually involves all the members of the implant team. The selection criteria may be considered in terms of age, cause of deafness, duration of severe or profound deafness, audiometric and vestibular assessment, otological and radiological examinations, general medical history, psychological profile and expectations. ➢ Congenitally deaf children derive significant benefit from cochlear implantation and constitute the largest group of children to receive cochlear implants.

		- Cochlear implantation process involves three major steps; selection, implantation and rehabilitation. The surgical procedure is not dissimilar to a mastoidectomy and is carried out under a general anaesthetic. The implant is switched on after the surgical wound has healed and programmed to individual requirement. - Serious complications following surgery are fortunately rare but could include implant hardware failure, infection including meningitis, facial nerve palsy and CSF leak.
97	K	Middle ear implant - Whilst a bone conduction hearing aid would be suitable, it is not the best option for this patient who required hearing whilst surfing. Middle ear implants are designed primarily for patients with moderate and severe sensorineural hearing loss, although with time they may be adapted for individuals with conductive or mixed hearing impairment. - The Symphonix Soundbridge system is made up of an external unit (comprising an audio processor, microphone and battery) and an

implantable component (consisting of a receiver coil, demodulator, conductor link wire and an electromagnetic floating mass transducer).

- The device is fitted surgically and the operation is similar to a mastoidectomy. The receiver is implanted into the skull just behind the ear. The external component is held on the side of the head by a magnet adjacent to the receiver and concealed behind the hairline.
- Sound energy is converted to a signal by the electronics in externally located audio processor and then transmitted to the internal electronic processing unit (receiver and demodulator). This sends an electrical signal, via the conductor link wire, to the electromagnetic floating mass transducer causing it to vibrate according to the frequency and amplitude of the original sound signal. The vibrations are directly transmitted to the incus in such a way as to mimic the true motion of the ossicles.
- The results so far with this new technology are very encouraging and

		patients have reported better quality sound than that provided by conventional aids.
98	N	Wilcoxon matched pairs test ➢ One group of subject (1 sample) who's perceived pain is recorded 1 day after surgery and 2 days after surgery (2 non parametric data sets). The test is named after Frank Wilcoxon (1892–1965) who proposed both this and the rank-sum test for two independent samples in 1945. ➢ The test was popularized by in 1956 by Siegel in his influential text book on non-parametric statistics. Siegel used the symbol T for the value defined below as S. Consequently, the test is sometimes referred to as the Wilcoxon t-test, and the test statistic is reported as a value of T. Other names may include the 't-test for matched pairs' or the 't-test for dependent samples'
99	C	Friedman Test ➢ This is used to detect differences in multiple treatments or in a treatment applied across multiple test attempts. The Friedman test is a non-parametric statistical test developed by the U.S. economist Milton

		Friedman. It is similar to the parametric repeated measures ANOVA. ➢ The procedure involves ranking each row (or block) together, then considering the values of ranks by columns. Applicable to complete block designs, it is thus a special case of the Durbin test. ➢ The Friedman test is used for one-way repeated measures analysis of variance by ranks. In its use of ranks it is similar to the Kruskal–Wallis one-way analysis of variance by rank. ➢ Friedman test is widely supported by many statistical software packages.
100	F	Man–Whitney U test ➢ In the study described in question 100, there is no ideal test, but the non-parametric Mann–Whitney makes the best use of the data and the least assumptions about the statistical properties of the pain scale. ➢ The Mann–Whitney U-test is use to compare two groups with respect to a non normal variable, and hence requires one variable to be binary (two-category) and one variable to be non normal measure. ➢ The next alternative similar test

		would be Kruskall–Wallis.

ND - #0106 - 060826 - C0 - 197/132/35 - PB - 9781784564186 - Gloss Lamination